D1172093

Stress Fractures

For Catherine

Stress Fractures

MICHAEL DEVAS F.R.C.S.

Consultant Orthopaedic Surgeon, Hastings
Research Assistant to the Orthopaedic Department
The Middlesex Hospital, London

CHURCHILL LIVINGSTONE
EDINBURGH LONDON AND NEW YORK
1975

Churchill Livingstone

Medical Division of Longman Group Limited

Distributed in the United States of America by
Longman Inc., New York, and by associated com-
panies, branches and representatives throughout the
world.

ISBN 0 443 01146 X

Library of Congress Catalog Card Number 74–78731

Printed in Great Britain

Preface

In 1957 the late Philip Wiles asked me to start the Stress Fracture Bureau at the Middle-sex Hospital; here were kept the records of patients with stress fractures. Many were collected by visiting various centres and perusing the records; as time went on many cases were sent to the bureau by colleagues not only from Great Britain but from all over the world. The ability of orthopaedic surgeons to co-operate with each other in research, irrespective of creed, colour or country, is to me one of the most encouraging signs that one day there will be a real international understanding and respect for all mankind. Also it must be obvious that the credit for any advances in the understanding of stress fractures made in this book go, not to me, but to all those who have sent me their cases. To me belong only the faults.

I have included in this book only those stress fractures of which I have records. The subject is still too young and too ill-understood to allow errors to be perpetuated by quotation. For example, I have seen no stress fractures of the neck of the fibula that might conform to the so-called parachutist's stress fracture. I do not know if that particular stress fracture exists but such fractures might equally well have been caused by violent muscle contraction on landing and not from repeated stress.

A close clinical study of stress and its effects on the living bone have influenced my thinking on other problems; so I believe, and I am not alone in this, that one cause of avascular necrosis is secondary to a compression stress fracture which has blocked off the blood supply.

The work is essentially clinical but without radiographs it is difficult to understand the effect of stress on bone; therefore the radiographs are in great profusion. Even so, the diagnosis of a stress fracture must be made clinically.

I offer this book as my sincere thanks to all my colleagues for their friendship in sending me cases. Some, lamentably, have died; others perhaps have been omitted through my inefficiency; to all I extend my gratitude; in particular it goes to the late Philip Wiles, and to Philip Newman, H. Jackson Burrows, Rodney Sweetnam, S. A. Jenkins, Christopher Attenborough, H. K. Bateman, Rodney Beals, A. Benjamin, G. Bentley, J. Bertram, A. C. Bingold, Eric Bintcliffe, Walter P. Blount, R. A. Bremner, D. R. Brothwell, John Buck, Norman Capener, Christopher Catterall, J. Crawford Adams, Paul H. Curtiss, David Cameron, P. J. Davidson, J. W. Dickson, F. Gaynor Evans, James Ellis, Jorgen Ernst, Maurice Fitzgerald, K. Franke, M. A. R. Freeman, R. H. Freeman, P. C. Fulford, Hoadley Gabb, R. W. Geise, H. C. Gjedde Jorgensen, George Glass, Eric Graham, P. F. Gray, R. Gruneberg, Robert Harris, M. H. M. Harrison, A. J. Harrold, D. E. Hastings, A. N. Henry, J. Hickman, A. R. Hodgson, J. K. Hooton, H. van der Houwen, M. Hunt, R. E. Irvine, N. E. James, B. V. Jones, E. W. Johnson, W. Kellock, Lipmann Kessel, I. Kessler, John Landells, Von B. Landgrot, W. A. Law,

John W. Leabhart, P. S. London, S. Mani, B. Sherwood Mather, Roy Maudsley, F. J. Milne, James Mills, H. L. McMullen, C. Nesbitt-Wood, G. Nesbitt-Wood, P. H. J. Nijs, Sir Henry Osmond-Clarke, P. H. Osterberg, Parisel-Leclercq, H. A. Pearce, H. Petty, A. H. C. Ratliff, Kenneth Reid, Robert Crawford-Robertson, Michael Robinson, James R. Rooney, David Ross, D. C. Sachdeva, R. H. Sewell, J. C. Scott, E. Shephard, L. A. H. Snowball, H. Graham Stack, F. G. St Clair Strange, Brian Thomas, D. Trevor, George X. Trimble, W. E. Tucker, H. S. Uberoi, L. C. Vaughan, O. Vaughan-Jackson, George P. Vose, G. J. Walley, Sir Reginald Watson-Jones, William Waugh, Ivan Williams, C. W. O. Windsor, F. T. Wheeldon.

This book would have had no value without good radiological reproductions, practically all of which were done by Mr M. Turney and his staff at the Photographic Department of the Middlesex Hospital; some of these radiographs have appeared in the *Journal of Bone and Joint Surgery* and are reproduced by kind permission of the editor and publishers. Last but by no means least, I thank the secretaries who have helped me to such a great extent, Miss Janet Cutmore, Mrs A. Caswell and Mrs E. Lilico.

1975   M. D.

Contents

CHAPTER ONE

INTRODUCTION

Stress fractures occur in the normal bones of healthy people doing everyday activities and with no injury. The type of stress fracture and the site at which it occurs in bone varies with age and activity. Most stress fractures heal with little treatment and no disfunction but some are not only disabling but dangerous. Fortunately these are few.

It is necessary to enlarge on the definition of a stress fracture. By normal is meant a person who has no disease and who, by everyday standards, is accepted as healthy. In this respect the bone of a child is different to that of a mature adult; with injury the bone may sustain a greenstick or a ripple fracture, neither of which are seen in the adult because the bone has changed with the normal process of ageing, to which all are subject; ageing, which varies from person to person, is accepted as a physiological and not as a pathological process. The fit 75-year-old is not so strong as in youth, but is nevertheless normal for that age. With the diminishing strength of muscle so does bone lose strength but is still normal for that age. This falling off of bone strength in the elderly, as with decubitus, is seen as osteoporosis and is not, in this context, a disease. This change is inevitable with longevity, and is a physiological process. Therefore stress fractures must, and do, vary from age to age, from the soft bone of children or the elderly to the tremendously strong bone of the mature adult.

Normal activity means that activity which any particular person might do leading a normal life. But the activity may not be usual. Thus the unaccustomed day's shopping in town is a normal activity for an ordinary woman in the same way that a championship race is normal for an athlete or a long march for a soldier. Very often in the history of a patient with a stress fracture the activity precipitating the fracture was unusual but must never have been abnormal.

The absence of injury is most important and any fracture that could have been caused by an injury has not been accepted as a stress fracture.

A healthy person hardly needs discussion but it is important to realise that stress fractures are common in athletes, that athletes are among the most fit of young people who are in the prime of life in any society; therefore it is not possible to consider that a person who has a stress fracture is unhealthy.

There are conditions which render patients more liable to fractures which are not caused by injury and follow the pattern of stress fractures but which lie outside the concept of the completely healthy person. For example, a person confined to a wheelchair, because of a painful osteoarthritis of the knees, may sustain a stress fracture of the ulna. Steroids used in the treatment of rheumatoid arthritis predispose to fractures that are identical to stress fractures in all other respects. These fractures are to be studied because they are of value to the knowledge of the subject as a whole.

A deformity in a limb is an abnormality but if the patient is otherwise normal it is permissible to study the stress fractures that occur with the different stress that is imposed on the bone concerned. Arthritis of the knee or hip seem to predispose to stress fractures, which, apart from the site, have all the other clinical features of a true stress fracture.

Perhaps the best-known stress fracture is the march fracture of the metatarsal bone (Fig. 1.1) but over the years stress fractures have been called by many different names of which pseudofractures, fatigue and spontaneous fractures are the most common. The term 'fatigue', although in some senses applicable, is misleading as it presupposes the pathology or biomechanics and suggests that bone, although a living tissue, will undergo the same molecular changes of fatigue as in metals and certain other inanimate substances. As yet, despite intense research, little is known about the reaction to stress of the living, as opposed to dead, bone which explains why the term stress fracture has come into use to describe this condition.

The pain of a stress fracture comes on at first after activity. It may be described as an ache, a stiffness, or even tiredness but always there is the relationship to activity (Fig. 1.2). If the activity is continued the pain comes on earlier each day until it prevents the exercise concerned. The ache will be present most of the day, but will go off eventually during the night. Thus, in the march fracture in a middle-aged woman, the pain first appears, perhaps, after a day's outing, and thereafter each day the pain comes on earlier during the day and, although relieved by rest, the patient will have to cut down her activity at which time she usually seeks advice.

SYMPTOMS AND SIGNS

The athlete who sustains a stress fracture will complain first of pain or aching around the site of the stress fracture which comes on after training or racing but passes off with rest. It recurs earlier the next day and with increased intensity. Within a further few days the pain occurs actually during training and ultimately is so severe that the athlete has to abandon his sport (Figs. 1.3 and 1.4). With this rest the pain soon lessens, but with premature resumption of training it returns worse than before. Any form of treatment, other than sufficient rest, has the same ill-effect of worsening the symptoms rapidly. Very occasionally pain comes on so severely and so quickly that an athlete cannot finish his sport; this is in contrast to the usual slow progress of the symptoms over several weeks. In retrospect the most important aspect of the symptoms is the recurrence of pain with exercise and the relief of pain with rest.

In the athlete, because of the normal rhythm required by training, the history is plain to all. With the ordinary patient the symptoms, although following a similar pattern, are not by any means so well defined because each day may have a different activity with a consequent alteration in the time or manner of the onset of the symptoms for each particular day.

The proper history will include the age, sex, everyday occupation and any untoward or unusual activity. All these facts may have a bearing on a stress fracture. It is again to be noted that the unusual activity must not be confused with an abnormal activity. Thus an athlete in training may usually run on a track but owing to exceptionally heavy rainfall he may have to train on a hard road instead. This is unusual but not abnormal and may precipitate a stress fracture. With athletics in particular, or any other activity in general, the methods used, the state of fitness, footwear, change in circumstances or even a holiday can be important. For example, the change from thick-soled rubber shoes to thin-soled track shoes with spikes may produce a stress fracture, or a recent holiday from home with extra walking will sometimes do the same.

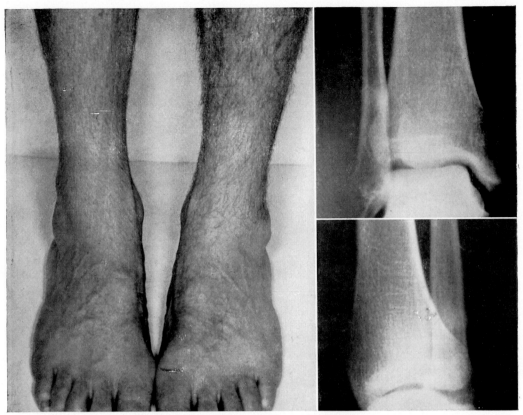

FIG. I.5   FIG. I.6

Only by comparing both ankles with the legs internally rotated can the swelling—caused by a stress fracture of the fibula—above the right lateral malleolus be seen with ease. The radiographs (Fig. I.6) show the stress fracture clearly five weeks after the onset of symptoms.

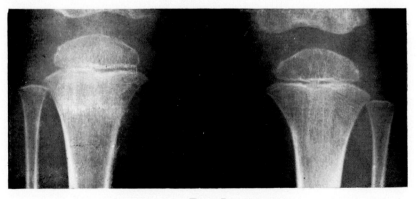

FIG. I.7

A boy of $3\frac{1}{2}$ was misdiagnosed as having a fractured femur when he complained of pain after stepping from a chair backwards. He was put into a plaster cylinder but when this was removed one month later the radiograph showed the haze of internal callus of a simple compression stress fracture of the upper third of the right tibia, from which he had made an excellent recovery with quite unnecessary treatment.

Compression stress fractures are seen particularly in children (Fig. 1.7) and in the older patient (Fig. 1.8). Certain bones only get compression stress fractures such as the calcaneus (Fig. 1.9). The neck of the femur (Fig. 1.10) and the tibia (Figs. 1.11 and 1.12) are sites at which compression stress fractures are common.

The distraction stress fracture has three main types. The most dangerous and fortunately the most rare is a transverse crack in one cortex of a long bone (Figs. 1.13 and 1.14), usually near its centre, which, with time and continued activity, breaks completely with all the morbidity of an ordinary fracture at that site. The commonest stress fracture is oblique, with a crack that runs through one cortex (Figs. 1.15 to 1.17); sometimes, as in the fibula (Figs. 1.3 and 1.4) or the metatarsal bones (Fig. 1.1), it becomes a complete fracture. The third type is a longitudinal stress fracture affecting a considerable length of the shaft of the bone concerned; it is, perhaps, an extension of an oblique crack, but seemingly from a different stress because it occurs at a different age (Figs. 1.18 and 1.19). Particularly they are seen in the tibia, the femur, the metatarsal bones and the fibula in children.

The distraction stress fractures are so called because, from radiological studies, it is apparent that the crack has started by the repeated bending of the bone away from the cortex in which the crack appears in much the same way that a bent stick breaks open with the crack first appearing on the convex side of the bend.

Some bones are subject only to tension; one example is the patella, which can have horizontal as well as vertical stress fractures.

The first radiological sign of a compression stress fracture is a faint haze or cloud within the confines of the cortices (Fig. 1.7). In serial radiographs this cloud is seen to develop into a mass of internal callus stretching across the bone; at this stage in some fractures the cortex is involved in the fracture (Fig. 1.20) and slight impaction or compression of the bone ends can occur. Eventually the fracture unites and the callus is absorbed. It leaves a permanent scar on the bone if there has been actual compression as sometimes occurs in the lower tibia in the elderly. It is rare for children who get compression stress fractures ever to show impaction or deformity, even when the periosteum is broken with the escape of callus beyond its confines. The time taken for a haze of new bone to appear in a compression fracture can be three months and occasionally longer, particularly in the calcaneus and lower tibia in adults.

The oblique stress fracture is the most common. It appears to start as a minute haze of new bone on the outer cortex of the bone which will not be seen if the radiograph is badly positioned or exposed (Fig. 1.21). The x-ray beam must pass tangentially to the affected cortical surface because it is only one small area that is first affected (Fig. 1.15). Gradually this callus increases and a small crack will appear in the cortex running obliquely across it, either proximally or distally, toward the medulla. The callus becomes more obvious and will be seen to encompass the fracture line in the cortex; often, by the time the latter is visible, union by callus is firm. Just occasionally the fracture shows very early; perhaps because the radiographer has had the good fortune to get the x-ray beam to pass squarely through the crack so that it is shown. The initial fracture at its onset is microscopical in size and it is only with time that it progresses sufficiently to show as a faint hairline crack, and then only with the best radiographic technique.

The positioning of the radiograph is particularly important in confirming the longitudinal stress fracture. In later stages it is seen as an area of callus passing along one

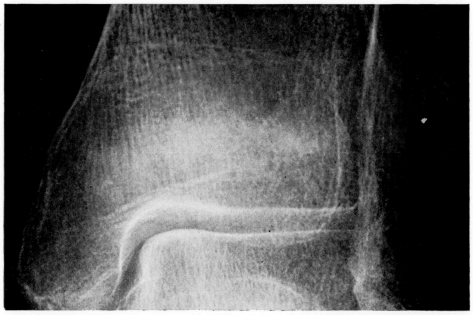

FIG. 1.8

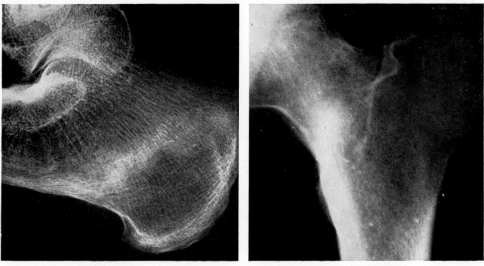

FIG. 1.9   FIG. 1.10

FIG. 1.8   A woman aged 78 developed pain in her left ankle which resisted diagnosis for many weeks until a slight haze of new bone within the lower tibia was found in the radiograph. This is a compression stress fracture of the lower end of the tibia.

FIG. 1.9   A woman of 47 developed pain in the heel which lasted many weeks before the radiograph confirmed the clinical diagnosis of a stress fracture of the calcaneus. This is a compression stress fracture and the line of the fracture follows the outline of the posterior surface of the tuberosity.

FIG. 1.10   A fat young woman of 18 developed pain in the hip which showed eventually in the radiograph as an area of increased density at the base of the neck. It was originally diagnosed as an osteoid osteoma. Tomographs eventually showed the fracture line, and the correct diagnosis was made. This particular form of stress fracture of the neck of the femur at this age does not usually displace.

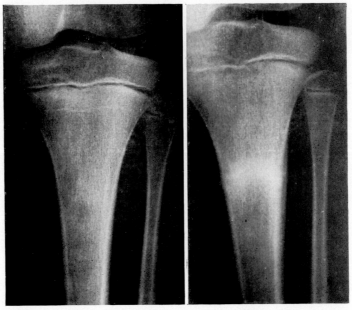

FIG. I.11   FIG. I.12

The presenting physical sign in a child was an ache in the upper shin. The first radiograph (Fig. I.11) was thought to show nothing abnormal but in the second (Fig. I.12), taken two weeks later, there is callus present shown as a haze passing across the shaft. In the earlier radiograph the very faint haze was then recognised. The second radiograph also shows that the lateral cortex has been breached and that there is a little callus under the periosteum outside the bone.

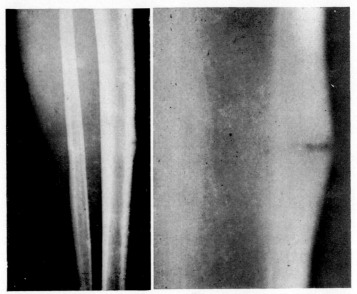

FIG. I.13   FIG. I.14

A college student of 19 played football and developed pain in the shins which was attributed to shin splints. Rapid running or forced use caused pain. Both legs became more painful. A radiograph was taken which showed, to the uninitiated, an innocuous-looking crack at the centre of the shaft. In the enlarged view (Fig. I.14) the crack is seen to extend right through one cortex. The opposite tibia had the same appearance. Failing to take the advice given he returned to football and broke the leg at the next game. This is a transverse stress fracture and is highly dangerous in this respect.

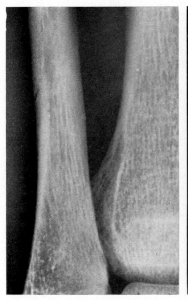 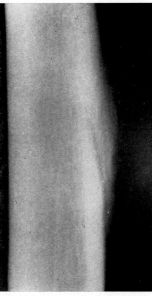

FIG. I.15   FIG. I.16

FIG. I.15

An athlete of 20 had had pain in the lower third of his left leg for five weeks before he was seen. Clinically there was swelling and tenderness over the lowermost third of the fibula and the radiograph shows clearly the stress fracture of the fibula.

FIG. I.16

A footballer aged 25 who played twice a week had had pain in his shin for two months; it had been strapped; when seen he was already getting better. He had pain and tenderness, particularly at the posteromedial aspect of the centre of the shaft of his tibia, where he had a high oblique stress fracture well shown in the radiograph.

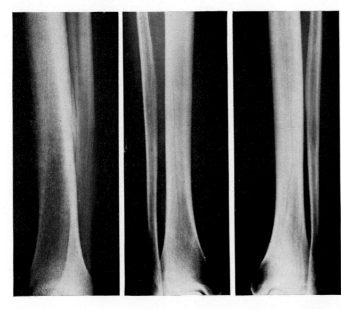

FIG. I.17   FIG. I.18   FIG. I.19

FIG. I.17

An athlete of 22 attended with a painful shin and there was a little tenderness and swelling to be felt. The radiograph shows what has in its time been called a 'periostitis' but this is an early stress fracture of the tibia.

FIG. I.18   FIG. I.19

A waitress was aged 61. She attended with pain and swelling in the left ankle for two months, having had no injury. This was now present all the time and kept her awake. The lower tibia was tender along the subcutaneous border and the radiographs showed it to have a longitudinal stress fracture which can be seen running a great distance up the shaft. Three months later she returned this time with similar symptoms in the right tibia which also had a longitudinal stress fracture.

B

surface of the cortex of a bone. With careful and painstaking radiography it can, at an earlier stage, be shown to be a long crack passing along one cortex and sometimes both (Figs. 1.18 and 1.19). Because of the great length of the fracture it does not show any tendency to deform or give way. Healing occurs, as shown by the callus on the surface of the cortical bone, but slowly. Usually at its distal end the longitudinal fracture line curves sharply to mimic the oblique stress fracture. Probably it is best not to consider that it is a more advanced form of the latter because there is a clinical difference between the two.

The small transverse crack, at right angles to the cortex, is the most ominous radiological sign of any stress fracture (Fig. 1.14). Uncommon, difficult to diagnose and treat, it can cause permanent disability because it allows the bone to break completely and to displace. The fracture, passing as it does straight across one cortex, soon weakens the bone; callus is slow to form; the crack increases in depth; the bone is now fragile and a slight jolt will break it. At first the crack is very small but the cortex above and below build up and pout out from the bone (Fig. 1.2). Callus, when it starts to form, is often divided at its centre in line with the fracture and continues thus because of the same stress that caused the initial lesion, so that it merely builds up the edges of the fracture without benefit of union. Any suspicion of this stress fracture calls for urgent action to prevent disaster.

The obvious radiological stress fracture, like any other lesion seen on a radiograph, must not be supposed to be the only one present; often stress fractures occur in more than one place with, perhaps, a second fracture at an earlier stage which may be missed (Figs. 1.22 and 1.23).

DIAGNOSIS

There are many systemic conditions that can cause local symptoms that might be mistaken for a stress fracture, and there are stress fractures that can be misdiagnosed as some other local, or general, disease.

The diagnosis of a stress fracture is dependent on the understanding of the history and clinical examination and on not expecting early radiological confirmation. No patient with a stress fracture will be misdiagnosed if the many varieties of the condition are known. Reliance must be placed on clinical judgement and not on confirmatory tests. It is the art of medicine at its best and not its science.

The differential diagnoses that may impinge at the site of any particular stress fracture are best considered when that specific fracture is studied; but certain general diseases must be considered in relation to stress fractures as a whole, such as rheumatoid arthritis and osteoarthritis.

General conditions that may be confused with stress fractures include the battered baby syndrome, which can be distinguished by the multiplicity of the injuries; infantile cortical hyperostosis, in which the hyperostosis on the tibia might possibly cause confusion, but again can be excluded by the typical changes elsewhere. Vitamin deficiencies, such as rickets or scurvy, are unlikely to cause difficulty because of the clinical appearance of the one and malaise of the other.

Low-grade fever in a child may accompany a stress fracture, and a subacute osteomyelitis may have to be excluded by the simple method of resting the child when the pain will cease and the spiky irregular pattern of the low fever will show that it is not infective in origin.

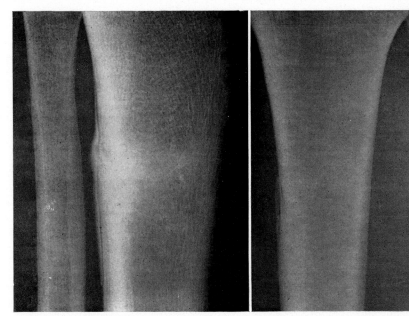

FIG. I.20

FIG. I.21

A boy of 12 attended hospital with pain, swelling and tenderness over the uppermost and middle thirds of the left tibia. The radiograph was reported as normal but, when compared with these later films, early periosteal reaction could be discerned in the posterior cortex. After two months he was quite better, having been treated by the avoidance of excess activity only.

An athlete of 31, who was a long-distance runner, had severe aching pain in both shins, intermittently, which had started a year previously. Running made it worse. It was worst in the uppermost third of the left tibia where there was tenderness; the radiograph shows an oblique stress fracture—but in the top of the tibia, so the fracture line passes downwards and outwards as compared to that in the lower part.

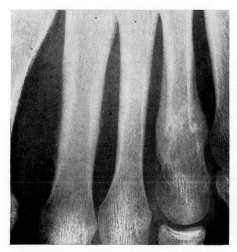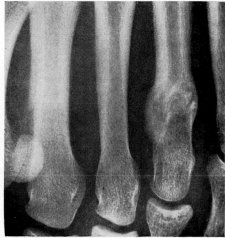

FIG. I.22

FIG. I.23

An athlete of 23 had had a stress fracture of the lower left fibula from which he had made a good recovery; four months later he attended with pain in the forefoot. He had developed two march fractures. That in the fourth metatarsal shaft is obvious but the other in the second metatarsal bone, which has only just started, is much less obvious.

In the young adult monarticular arthritis, whether rheumatoid or infective, causes slight difficulty only; tenosynovitis as a presenting lesion in collagen disease or from a local pathology can give pain and swelling that may simulate that of a stress fracture; the examination and a knowledge of anatomy will dispel any misapprehension in this respect.

As age increases, gout and pseudogout become more apparent and in the foot may be quite difficult to exclude. The failure of rest to relieve the pain and the low threshold of stimulation necessary to produce the pain are helpful. It must not be forgotten that a stress fracture may precipitate an exacerbation of gout, for the latter, hyena-like, prefers to attack an injured part. Gouty deposits in tendons, such as the calcaneal, induce rupture which, if insidious, causes pain that is worse with exercise; if the examination is not careless this should not confuse.

Vascular disease, from varicose veins to intermittent claudication, may give symptoms or signs that suggest stress fractures; the new bone formed by a stress fracture has been attributed to overlying varicosities.

Local lesions that can occur at any site include inflammation of the skin, stings, fat necrosis, neurolipomata and other painful soft tissue tumours; all have been inculpated as the cause of the symptoms of a stress fracture.

Primary neoplasms, again especially in children, can be the most worrying differential diagnosis, but the speed of progress of a stress fracture in a child often dispels any doubt even before a biopsy can be arranged. An osteoid osteoma, with its different pattern of symptoms, is not difficult to exclude except radiologically when the thickened cortex of one side of a bone may mislead, especially if the central nidus is thought to be the fracture line. Failure to achieve relief by rest will soon throw doubt on the diagnosis of a stress fracture. A bone weakened by a neoplasm will often give exactly the same symptoms as a stress fracture because the weakened bone does, in fact, slowly fracture until the overt pathological fracture occurs.

A small warning is necessary in the interpretation of radiography. A nutrient artery can, at times, be seen as a classical oblique stress fracture and, as a result, the correct diagnosis is missed.

TREATMENT

The best treatment for all stress fractures is rest from any activity that causes the pain. If activity is continued, the pain will get worse until the patient cannot go on, whether at work or sport. With insufficient rest the symptoms recur with redoubled intensity, particularly in the athlete.

The normal treatment of a patient with a stress fracture is ambulatory. An elastic adhesive bandage is sufficient for nearly all stress fractures of the lower leg. For other fractures partial relief of weight-bearing by the use of crutches or a walking frame—according to the age and capabilities of the patient—are also indicated. The advice to some athletes to rest from sport has to be enforced by using a plaster cast to ensure that the rest is taken.

Certain stress fractures, such as in the neck of the femur, in the midshaft of the tibia or transversely in the patella need immediate admission to hospital for treatment, which may necessitate open operation and internal fixation.

The worst advice of all is to tell the patient to disregard the symptoms; to run it off; to have it manipulated or to inject it with locally acting steroids.

PREVENTION OF STRESS FRACTURES

This is important to the athlete in whom stress fractures occur more during intense training than in maintaining fitness because the strength of bone lags behind the increase in muscle power; in part this may be caused by newer ways of achieving fitness in which will-power plays a great part in sustained and extreme muscular effort. Therefore, the athlete must train steadily and progressively. A sudden change of training, such as from a soft track to a hard road, must be taken carefully. Thick, soft-soled shoes can compensate for the hardness of the road.

People other than athletes, and especially the middle-aged, develop stress fractures after doing something unusual but not abnormal at work or at leisure. Thus staying with relations who live on a rough road, a holiday in a hilly town or a walking tour can cause a stress fracture; it is impossible to advise perpetual abstinence from such excursions as a preventative, although good shoes and ample rest may help. In the older patient with idiopathic osteoporosis decubitus is to be avoided because activity maintains muscle tone and muscle tone maintains the strength of bone.

AETIOLOGY

Accurate statistics on the occurrence of stress fractures are difficult to obtain except from a particular centre which may give its own findings for one or another type of patient, as, for example, a military hospital which has to deal with many recruits. Certainly the experience of the Stress Fracture Bureau cannot be used for general statistics in the occurrence of stress fractures because, with time, the more difficult and abstruse stress fractures were being included in higher proportions and do not represent the average rate of occurrence.

Despite this, certain points arise: athletics in any form produce stress fractures in healthy young adults; age has a similar effect with, in particular, the femoral neck at risk; children, barely old enough to walk, break, with no injury, their fibula or tibia. At any age the normal bone has, with normal use, fractured from the stresses of every-day activity.

The cause of a stress fracture is muscular pull; it is not the jarring of the foot landing on the ground. The fibula is not a weight-bearing bone yet it often sustains stress fractures; they also occur in the arm especially in certain athletics; here without doubt there is no weight-bearing. Muscle pull will bend the normal bone. Simple contraction of the calf muscles can draw the fibula towards the tibia and, in like manner, though more difficult to demonstrate, the tibia towards the fibula. A simple experiment demonstrates this. With the subject sitting the leg is put into a wooden frame (Fig. 1.24) and two radiographs taken on the same plate, first with the leg relaxed, the second with the calf muscles attempting full flexion against the resistance of the frame. The developed plate will then show that the outline of the tibia and the lateral malleolus fit accurately but that the shaft of the fibula has cast a double image, indicating that it has been moved towards the tibia by the contracture of the muscles (Fig. 1.25).

It is clear that in normal running the contracture of all muscles in the calf to flex the ankle or to resist its extension will pull the fibula and tibia towards each other; the more forceful the contraction the greater the movement of the fibula towards the tibia and the greater the stress imposed upon it, especially at the junction of the shaft with the firmly fixed lateral malleolus, which is where most of the fractures occur. This in part explains why there is an increase in fractures with a change from soft to

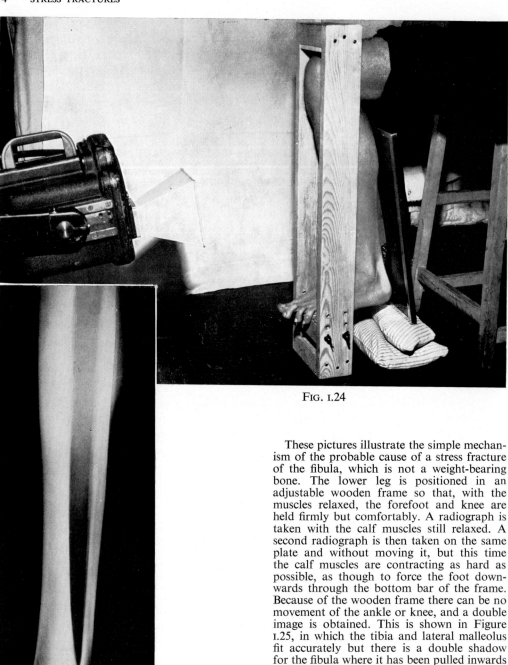

FIG. 1.24

FIG. 1.25

These pictures illustrate the simple mechanism of the probable cause of a stress fracture of the fibula, which is not a weight-bearing bone. The lower leg is positioned in an adjustable wooden frame so that, with the muscles relaxed, the forefoot and knee are held firmly but comfortably. A radiograph is taken with the calf muscles still relaxed. A second radiograph is then taken on the same plate and without moving it, but this time the calf muscles are contracting as hard as possible, as though to force the foot downwards through the bottom bar of the frame. Because of the wooden frame there can be no movement of the ankle or knee, and a double image is obtained. This is shown in Figure 1.25, in which the tibia and lateral malleolus fit accurately but there is a double shadow for the fibula where it has been pulled inwards towards the tibia. The contracting muscles, attached to both tibia and fibula, cause approximation of the two bones because of the resultant of the forces that are produced.

The commonest site for the stress fracture in the fibula is just above the lateral malleolus where the greatest bend appears to have taken place in this simple experiment.

hard ground or from gentle to intensive training. It must be emphasised that it is not the foot landing on the ground that causes a stress fracture but the muscle contracture that resists the weight of the body passing through the various bones of the leg to the ball of the foot. If the runner landed on the ball of his foot with no contraction of his muscles the ankle would immediately extend and the heel would hit the ground with a painful jar.

That the muscle contraction causes the fracture is also shown in the calcaneus. This does not get its compression stress fracture by the banging of the heel on the ground in marching or walking, but by the compression that is caused by the result—or moment—of the force that occurs within the bone from the two opposite forces that go to it, the first from the calf muscles contracting and pulling on the tuberosity of the calcaneus through the calcaneal tendon and the second, resisting this force, being the long plantar ligaments attached to the tuberosity. The resultant of the force passes towards the ankle; therefore, the compression stress fracture should occur at right angles to the line joining any particular part of the posterior aspect of the tuberosity of the calcaneus to the ankle joint. This is usually what is found clinically. This principle is well shown in Figures 1.26 to 1.29. First, in Figures 1.26 and 1.27, is shown the calcaneus of a boy who fell from the roof of a shed and landed on his heels. He was suspected of having sustained a fracture of the calcaneus but nothing showed on the original radiographs. Three weeks later, however, a line of new bone formation within the calcaneus could be seen but this was running parallel to the plantar surface of the foot. When the boy landed on his heel the force went directly upwards through the bone, slightly compressing it and causing this fracture which, although caused by injury, resembles the internal callus of a stress fracture. A second demonstration of the force necessary to produce the type of lesion seen in a stress fracture is shown in Figure 1.28. This particular fracture was caused by a man kick-starting a motor mower. He pressed the starting pedal down forcefully with the ball of his foot but the machine backfired, and the pedal came back forcefully. The calf muscles were contracting powerfully at the time of the backfire when there was a sudden increase in resistance by the pedal attempting to extend the foot and ankle. Thus a large amount of force was transmitted through the calcaneus as a result of the moment of the forces pulling upon it from the calf and forwards from it in the direction of the long plantar ligament. An immediate traumatic compression fracture was caused. When this illustration is compared to Figure 1.29, which is of a straightforward compression stress fracture, the similarity of the site and direction of the fracture is at once apparent.

The pattern of stress fractures alters with age; the child and a healthy old person often share the same type. Old age weakens generally, muscle tone is reduced, the bones lose calcium. Perhaps this is why the similarity exists.

Stress fractures other than in the limbs are rare with the exception of the ribs in which they were particularly common after thoracoplasty. But the cases that are still seen, especially in children, may cause anxiety in diagnosis because of a vague resemblance to a tumour.

The underlying cause of a stress fracture is not difficult to understand with good clinical observation; perhaps too much emphasis has been put on scientific testing of bone strength, which has mostly been on dead bone from which the living bone is as different as the proverbial cheese from chalk.

The normal healthy adult in the prime of life develops, in a normal bone, a stress fracture. This fracture occurs with normal activity. Often this is intense and needing much muscular energy. Strong muscles need strong bones. If a stress fracture occurs the skeleton is taking greater stress than that for which it is ready. We are left with the paradox that the normal use of the body will cause a normal bone to break; not necessarily suddenly, but slowly and insidiously. The first that can be seen of a stress fracture in the radiograph is a minute crack. Symptoms will have preceded this by varying periods of time. Therefore, the crack must have started as a smaller crack; it is possible to work back in this way and to postulate that a stress fracture starts at molecular level and not as the sudden appearance of a macroscopic break as if it really was a 'spontaneous' fracture.

At molecular level we find that the hardness of bone is imparted by the apatite crystal; the durability by the collagen fibres. The latter are not rigid and will break only if they are encased in a rigid material that breaks, otherwise the collagen will bend.

The apatite crystal is therefore suspect. The blood supply to a bone in the healthy adult is considerable and for a purpose, because Nature does not squander her resources. If the living bone has this rich blood supply it needs it. When a bone is used the energy absorbed by the bone in resisting the stresses and strains that are put upon it must be dissipated; this would best be done by a denaturing of the apatite crystalline structure. Only by the blood supply can the apatite crystals be refreshed so that it may again become an integral part in the strength of the bone as a whole.

The greater the use of a limb, the greater the strength of a bone. This is well known in orthopaedic practice. No patient in a plaster is allowed to lie immobile but continued use of all parts not immobilised and use of the immobilised part as a whole is insisted upon, for otherwise severe decalcification of the bone occurs. No bone, therefore, will remain stronger than it need be to resist the everyday stresses and strains that occur within it. Nature, as it were, sees no need for a strong and rigid bone in a weak and unused limb.

The same problem is now being met in space travel, in which weightlessness is an advanced form of absolute decubitus, and so it will not be surprising if astronauts, after a long weightless voyage, develop stress fractures on return to earth.

In order to strengthen a bone decalcified by disuse the musculature around it must be used. The muscles must increase in tone, and it is use, or activity, that is the basic necessity in building up bone so that it becomes strong enough to accept the increased stress: but this strength of the bone as a whole is achieved by increased strength at molecular level.

It is acceptable to assume that the normal person will use such exertion as is needed and that the denaturing of the apatite crystal is offset by other crystals being refreshed. When the denaturing exceeds the refreshment a point is reached at which actual collapse of apatite crystals occurs to an extent that is pathological rather than molecular and which allows the blood to escape from the vessels within the bone, which at once must cause a physical inflammatory process. Once this has started, local resorption of bone occurs, the blood supply increases, further local weakening of the bone and further resorption stimulate new blood vessels to penetrate and rebuild the local structure of the bone. As soon as this pathological change has started at cellular level its onward progress is assured with continuing activity stressing further the slightly weakened area, in the same way that a crack in a plate-glass window will continue inexorably to progress with the vibration of the nearby traffic.

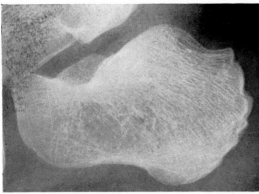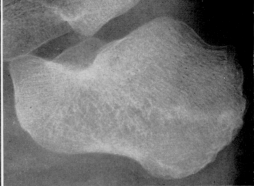

FIG. I.26	FIG. I.27

A boy fell from the roof of a shed and landed on his heels. The symptoms suggested a fracture of the calcaneus, but the first radiograph was normal (Fig. I.26). Three weeks later a traumatic compression fracture can be seen quite clearly (Fig. I.27), but the direction of the internal callus is quite different from that in a compression stress fracture, for here it runs horizontally and at right angles to the line of force that caused the fracture.

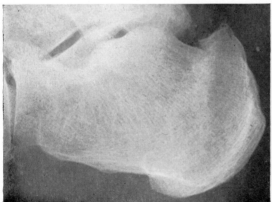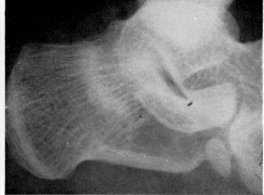

FIG. I.28	FIG. I.29

A man aged 49 was kick-starting a motor mower when it backfired. The pedal under the ball of the foot forced the ankle into extension against the resistance of his calf muscles. The radiograph shows a fracture, with some displacement, but following the line of a compression stress fracture, caused by this violence transmitted through the long plantar ligament in one direction and resisted by the calcaneal tendon and its muscles in the other. It is this mechanism that causes the compression stress fracture in this bone that occurs in marching or walking.

This is the radiograph of a man who sustained a classical stress fracture of his calcaneus. Notice the curve of the internal callus in quite a different direction to the callus of the boy in Figure I.26 above although the direction corresponds with the fracture in Figure I.28.

Stress fractures and osteoporosis pose a difficult problem. It is much more common to find stress fractures in women over the age of 50 than in men of similar age, and undoubtedly this has a connection with idiopathic or postmenopausal osteoporosis. But it is not possible to say that all women over the age of 50 are abnormal; it is permissible to allow some slight degree of osteoporosis as compatible with the normal health of women over the menopause.

Stress fractures in women over the age of 50 are identical in all respects to other stress fractures. For example, the stress fractures of the lowest third of the fibula in an athlete is exactly the same as that which occurs in the middle-aged woman. So we have a paradox; the athlete is physically fit and could not be a better example of the normal in physique (unless it is to be supposed that he is better than normal, or a 'superman' physiologically), yet athletes and middle-aged women get the same stress fracture. Here it has been accepted that mild osteoporosis is not pathological and that it is part of the normal process of ageing for the person concerned. The stress fractures that occur in middle age are entirely consistent with all other stress fractures and to exclude the stress fracture in women over 50 would be wrong.

CHAPTER TWO

STRESS FRACTURES OF THE FIBULA

Stress fractures of the fibula occur at any age and, as a whole, are found equally in both sexes although at different ages; young men and boys have a slight preponderance because of their interest in athletics. In middle age and in the elderly it is more common in women.

The stress fracture of the fibula is usually in its lowest third; less often, except in children, the fracture is higher up. It is usual for symptoms to start insidiously but occasionally the onset is abrupt; a mild ache in the ankle may precede a sudden exacerbation of symptoms. The fractures are often bilateral, but with a time interval of a few months to a year between the two fractures perhaps because, as with other stress fractures, the decrease in activity imposed by the most advanced and painful fracture prevents the opposite side from progressing or causing symptoms.

A typical stress fracture of the fibula is found just above the lateral malleolus and occurs after a period of increased activity or, in the case of athletics, intensive training or sport. The history is straightforward: at first aching after use, then during use perhaps with a severe exacerbation of pain which often causes the patient to seek advice. A swelling of the outer ankle may have been noticed. Finally the aching is severe, continuous and interferes with sleep.

An example of the development of a stress fracture of the lowest third of the fibula is shown in Figures II.1 to II.4, which are the radiographs of a middle-aged woman who had walked more than usual. At first only the lateral cortex appears to have been involved but the last radiograph shows that both cortices ultimately are fractured.

Stress fractures of the fibula can be divided into those occurring in childhood, in athletes or young adults, in middle age and, finally, in the elderly in whom often it is associated with a stress fracture of the tibia; sometimes these double stress fractures are in the uppermost third of the bones just below the knee. They are considered in Chapter Four. The 'parachutist's' stress fracture of the neck of the fibula has not been seen. The stress fracture of the fibula in athletes has also been called the runner's fracture. A study of this gives a good introduction to the understanding of stress fractures.

The Runner's Fracture

Stress fractures of the fibula in young adults or athletes are usually in the lower part of the fibula some 3 to 7 cm above the tip of the lateral malleolus; in about 25 per cent of patients the fracture is higher up the shaft. The athletes are in the full vigour of youth and are fit in all other respects. They are specially liable to this fracture if they overexercise when not in training or suddenly alter their methods. New recruits to military service are also susceptible to this fracture. Nonetheless, the fractures also occur in full training or in actual races.

19

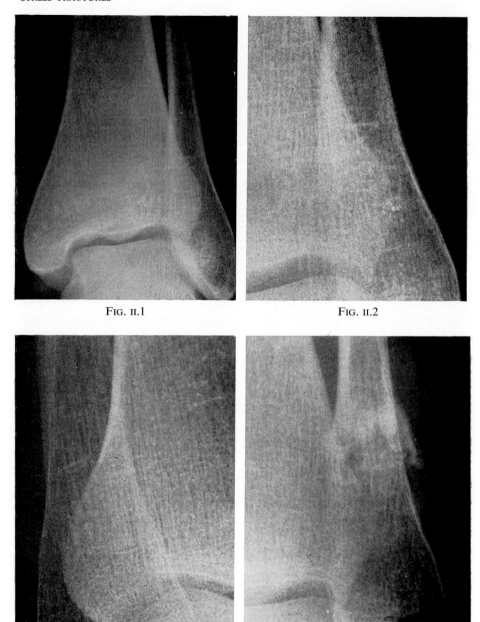

FIG. II.1   FIG. II.2

FIG. II.3   FIG. II.4

These radiographs show how a stress fracture of the fibula may present in radiographs. They are of a middle-aged woman who had walked more than usual and who attended with pain in the left ankle that had started insidiously some two or three weeks before. In Figure II.1 the fracture line is almost invisible but could be seen in the original radiograph when it was held to a naked light. However, the enlarged view of that radiograph in Figure II.2 does show a small crack, just above the Harris line, which runs upwards and inwards in the lateral cortex of the fibula. The lateral view (Fig. II.3), taken at the same time, is normal even in the enlargement. The radiograph in Figure II.4, taken just over eight weeks later, shows the stress fracture, which runs up through the cortex on the outer side and then across the bone to make the fracture complete. The external callus is well shown, as is the callus across the lower fibula shaft.

SYMPTOMS AND SIGNS

The athlete presents with a complaint of two or three weeks pain and aching in the outer ankle which started insidiously (Fig. II.5). The sudden onset of symptoms is a less common finding but often there has been a sudden exacerbation of the pain which indicates that either a partial fracture has become complete and that the mild preceding symptoms passed unnoticed until that moment or that the stress fracture is higher than usual.

It is not usual for the athlete to recall a particular moment when the symptoms started; instead, an aching gradually became noticeable during, or just after, activity. Often said to be behind the ankle, a tender spot may have been found well to the back of the ankle bone or lateral malleolus. With time, the pain comes on earlier during training and persists longer with rest until eventually the sport has to be stopped. By now, any sudden movement will cause pain, and a swelling may have been noticed above the lateral malleolus (Fig. II.7 and II.8). Walking is possible with a greater or lesser degree of limp and pain, or with none, but running, jumping onto a bus or similar activity hurts. There may be a history of a previous stress fracture.

It is usual for the athlete to associate the symptoms with increased or altered activity in early training. One form of increased activity localised to the leg is the change from running on soft ground to a hard road or track.

Inspection of the ankle may show a swelling of the lower fibula but it is not easy to see. Often the local swelling on the fibula is entirely masked by slight general swelling of the ankle. Only by very careful comparison with the eye level with the ankle and with the feet rotated inwards can the local swelling on the fibula be seen. If the fracture is at one of the less common sites higher up the shaft nothing can be seen.

The examining hand is a very much more delicate instrument than the eye for this fracture and a swelling may be felt under the skin over the fracture site on the subcutaneous border of the fibula. This swelling, although soft and tender at first, becomes bony hard in time and the top and the bottom margins blend in to the shaft of the fibula and at its front and back it disappears under the neighbouring soft tissues. Although the swelling can be felt quite early in the condition it is important to remember that it is not necessarily visible radiologically, however hard it feels.

Pressure over the swelling causes considerable pain, and pressure over the upper shaft of the fibula or 'springing' it may cause pain at the fracture site. Movements of the knee and ankle will be free as will be those of the foot but certain muscular effort will cause the pain; particularly does flexion of the ankle and foot against resistance as in standing on tiptoe. Forced inversion or eversion of the talus to move the lateral malleolus may sometimes cause the pain but this is not necessarily so because of the very strong lower tibiofibular ligaments.

RADIOGRAPHY

It is a general rule that the radiological confirmation of stress fractures is late, and those of the fibula are no exception. Several weeks may pass before the fracture shows in the radiograph, during which time neither must the clinical diagnosis be discarded nor the athlete allowed to start training. A very slight haze of periosteal new bone on the posterolateral aspect of the fibula may be the first change in the radiograph, as is shown in Figures II.9 to II.11. It took six weeks for the fracture to show clearly. Another finding in the radiograph may be of a very slight haze of new bone clouding the shaft

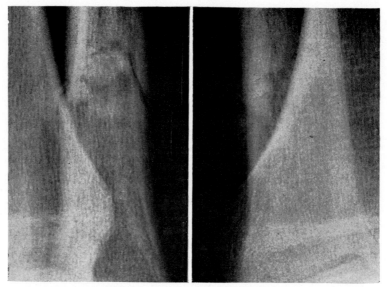

FIG. II.5   FIG. II.6

A cross-country runner had had pain for three weeks in the region of the left lateral malleolus. It was strapped by his general practitioner, which helped, but the athlete felt a lump under the strapping and, worried, sought further attention. On close questioning he said that he had been running in a four mile race on a road and at three and a quarter miles felt the slight onset of pain which slowly got worse. Before this he had been training on a cinder track and across country. He had worn thin-soled plimsolls for his road running, but track spikes in the country. He had tried to 'run the pain off' but this made it worse. The first radiographs at three weeks show the typical line of the fracture running through the outer cortex of the fibula, with the fracture extending medially across the shaft with early callus formation. When the fibula is approximated to the tibia by the muscles this would tend to open this crack.

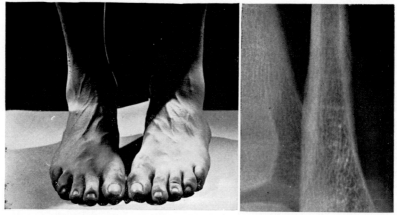

FIG. II.7   FIG. II.8

A cross-country runner aged 23 had had pain in his left ankle for one week. It was particularly painful on walking and was eased by rest. He had already noticed a slight but hard swelling above his ankle, which is shown in the clinical photograph (Fig. II.7). It is very difficult to see the swelling of a stress fracture even in subcutaneous bones, and the examining hand is better than the eye. Careful comparison of the ankles by medially rotating the legs is always necessary. This particular athlete had been doing road training in thin-soled shoes and had alternated fast and slow running over every 100 yards. Figure II.8 is a radiograph of the stress fracture; four months later he developed two march fractures (Figs. I.22 and I.23, p. 11).

of the fibula just above the malleolus, but it may take four weeks or more to show. In Figure II.12 is shown a radiograph four weeks after the onset of symptoms. The radiograph two weeks after the start of symptoms did show slight abnormality but this was insufficient to show in a reproduction. It was only at four weeks that the stress fracture was obvious.

The earliest changes are often seen only if the radiograph is held to a naked bulb, even on a properly exposed radiograph, because, of necessity, the affected part of the fibula is 'overexposed' in the normal method of radiography of the ankle. Figure II.13 shows the changes at nine weeks, at which time the fracture line could be seen for the first time even though slight new bone formation had been visible a little earlier. Unless the radiographs are repeated, sometimes after the symptoms have ceased, the actual fracture line may never be seen.

The stress fracture starts at the posterolateral aspect of the fibula, on average 5 cm above the tip of the lateral malleolus. When the crack can be seen, it runs proximally and medially through the outer cortex of the fibula from the posterolateral aspect and across the shaft in an irregular horizontal direction. The stress fracture starts as the small oblique crack in the outer cortex and the bone, thus weakened, breaks completely; if this occurs suddenly it will give rise to the severe or abrupt onset of symptoms of which some patients complain.

Aids to radiographic diagnosis should not be necessary if good exposures are made on carefully positioned plates. The normal anteroposterior and lateral views are not always sufficient to show the lesion to its best advantage; oblique views may show callus formation when otherwise it might not be seen (Figs. II.14 and II.15). Very rarely a macrograph may help (Figs. II.16 and II.17), with which the fracture may be seen earlier than in the ordinary radiographs. It is very important to remember that a hairline crack in the cortex of a bone will only be seen if the x-ray beam passes through the plane of the fracture. If it is above or below this plane the hairline fracture will not show. Thus it is of value in ordering radiographs to mark the exact spot at which it is thought the fracture has occurred.

DIAGNOSIS

The typical history of pain starting insidiously at the outer side of the ankle and continuing to get worse with activity so that ultimately sport has to stop, combined with rest pain, particularly in the evening, is sufficient to cause suspicion.

The examination will always reveal tenderness, usually just above the lateral malleolus; and pain can sometimes be elicited by springing the fibula, and swelling is present on the fibula if the fracture is in the lowest third of the fibula but, because often there is a slight general swelling of the ankle, it cannot always be seen. At first the swelling on the fibula is soft and very tender and it gradually becomes hard with healing.

The shaft of the fibula sustains stress fractures but accounts for only a quarter of those seen in the fibula in athletes. Figures II.18 and II.19 show a high, long, oblique stress fracture that was first seen radiologically at four weeks. This fracture remained incomplete, as is shown by the lack of callus medially and the sound healing on the lateral aspect at 12 weeks. Figure II.20 shows a similar but complete fracture that occurred in a marathon runner, in full training, who felt a sudden pain in his leg at the 22nd mile. He was adamant that he had not injured himself in any way and that he had felt no pain previously.

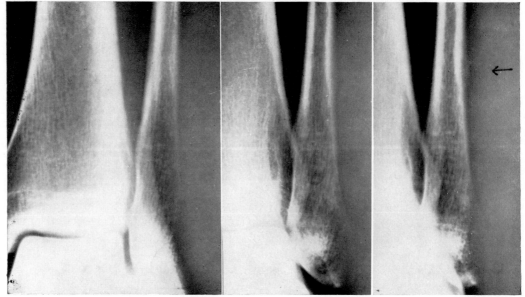

FIG. II.9   FIG. II.10   FIG. II.11

The radiographic confirmation of a stress fracture is late. In Figure II.9 there is no abnormality to be seen 10 days after the onset of symptoms in an athlete; in Figure II.10, four weeks later, the changes are just visible as a slight periosteal haze of new bone but so faint as to be difficult to reproduce. However, at six weeks, in Figure II.11 the new bone at the fracture site is more clear.

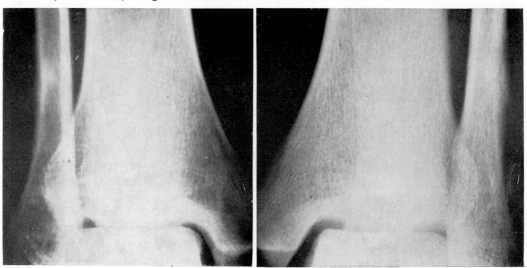

FIG. II.12   FIG. II.13

To emphasise how difficult it is to see the stress fracture, Figure II.12 shows the radiograph of an athlete four weeks after the occurrence of symptoms. The stress fracture can just be seen; two weeks previously the radiograph seemed entirely normal until it was inspected against the naked light of an unscreened bulb. Only then was a very slight periosteal reaction visible, too slight to be seen in reproduction.

Sometimes the stress fracture is not only slow to show radiologically but may also be very slight. If radiographs are not taken at regular intervals the diagnosis may never be confirmed. The radiograph of the athlete shown in Figure II.13 was taken nine weeks after the onset of symptoms and it was only at this late stage that the fracture was seen as such, there having been a little haze of new bone formation previously.

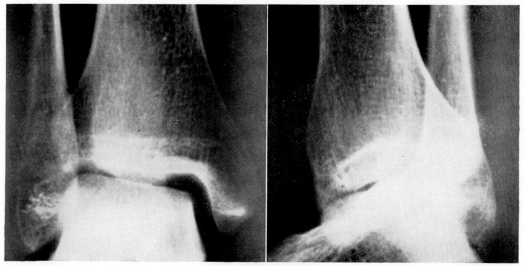

FIG. II.14   FIG. II.15

In order to confirm a stress fracture the ordinary anteroposterior and lateral radiographs should, if they are normal, be supplemented by oblique views. Figure II.15 shows the very small mass of new bone on the posterolateral aspect of the upper part of the lateral malleolus which did not show in the normal anteroposterior (Fig. II.14) and lateral views.

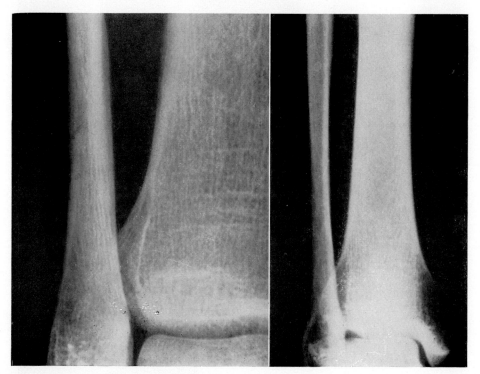

FIG. II.16   FIG. II.17

A well-centred macrograph may show a crack in a bone earlier than can be seen in the ordinary radiograph. Figure II.16 shows such a crack which was not seen in the normal radiograph (Fig. II.17). Both figures are reproduced in relative sizes.

C

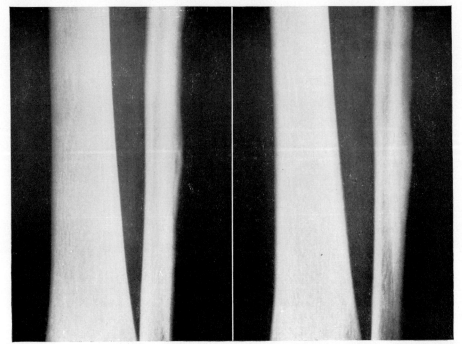

FIG. II.18   FIG. II.19

FIG. II.18   FIG. II.19

A stress fracture of the shaft of the fibula
in which the fracture line can hardly be seen
in the reproduction (Fig. II.18) but in the
original radiograph it was visible running
beneath the callus very obliquely upwards
through the lateral cortex of the fibula. Two
months later the fracture had completely
healed radiologically (Fig. II.19) with only a
slight bump on the lateral cortex to indicate
where it had been.

FIG. II.20

Another long, oblique stress fracture of the
shaft of the fibula is shown in this radiograph
of a marathon runner who was aged 38. This
fracture occurred in his 22nd mile and he was
adamant there had been no injury or previous
pain. The unusual direction of the fracture and
its length is well shown.

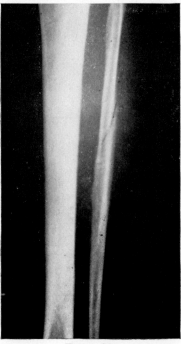

FIG. II.20

The differential diagnosis of a stress fracture of the fibula in an athlete must include other local injuries, such as a muscle violence fracture (Figs. II.21 and II.22), tenosynovitis and an insidious rupture of the calcaneal tendon. All can be excluded by the examination. It is unlikely that systemic conditions will cause difficulty in the athlete. The greatest danger is not to consider a stress fracture because of no radiological confirmation. A stress fracture diagnosed and treated early may heal without the fracture ever being visible in the radiograph.

The fracture that occurs with an abrupt onset, or when there has been an acute episode on top of symptoms that started insidiously, is usually quicker to be seen radiologically because the fracture has become complete suddenly and some minute displacement will allow the crack to show. This is well seen in the radiographs in Figures II.23 and II.24 which are of an athlete who had sustained a complete stress fracture across the fibula just above the lateral malleolus. This particular fracture is one of the lowest that occurs in the fibula.

TREATMENT

It is most important to obtain the confidence of the athlete in the diagnosis and the necessity for treatment; he is usually reluctant to give up sport or training, particularly if there is the chance of participation in an important event: the advice to rest is highly distasteful. A careful explanation that the bone is broken and it must be allowed to unite firmly also causes disquiet. The reason for the break must be explained and it must also be made clear that, after the bone has united, it will require strengthening by graduated activity. When training is restarted there must be a careful watch; any recurrence of symptoms indicates more rest. Once this principle of rest has been accepted simple elastic adhesive bandages will normally be sufficient especially for the recreational athlete.

For the professional athlete it is sometimes necessary to use a plaster-of-Paris cast below the knee, on which the patient can walk, mostly to curb any enthusiasm to try out the ankle too soon. The elastic adhesive strapping must be applied by the surgeon and not left to a nurse. Using a roll three inches wide, it should be applied from the metatarsal heads to well up to the calf. Starting over the fifth metatarsal bone, the strapping is applied medially across the dorsum of the foot, under the ball of the foot and then it sweeps round proximally up and across to the medial malleolus, behind the ankle, round the lateral malleolus and down in a figure of eight to the medial border of the forefoot, each layer overlapping to leave about 2 cm of the previous layer exposed. This gives firm support with the outer side of the foot pulled upwards, or proximally, with each sweep of the strapping across the dorsum of the foot and around the medial malleolus. One roll applied in this way is usually sufficient and the immediate relief of pain indicates that it has been properly applied; this gives the athlete the final touch of confidence in the medical adviser. Far too often, the athlete, through lack of confidence, fails to follow advice, not only with this fracture but also with those at other sites, and then by training too soon has to be off sport much longer than might have been necessary.

General fitness must be maintained by exercising. This must be done cautiously, but without causing pain in the ankle and so that no other lesion is produced, and overuse of the opposite leg must be avoided (Figs. II.25 and II.26).

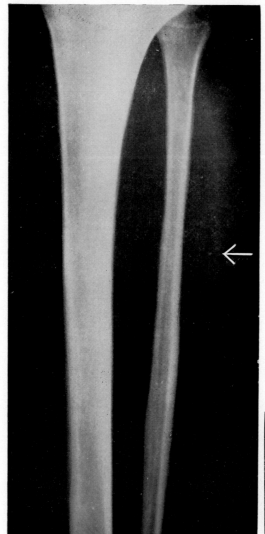

FIG. II.21

Stress fractures must always be very carefully differentiated from muscle violence
causing a fracture by a forceful and awkward
movement. Figure II.21 shows what at first
appeared to be a normal fibula but the footballer concerned said that he had made an
awkward kick with great force which had
immediately produced a severe pain in the
calf. The arrow marks the site of tenderness
at that time (Fig. II.21). Two weeks later a
slight haze of periosteal new bone was seen
on the medial side of the fibula. This was
much clearer four weeks later (Fig. II.22).
This is not a stress fracture but the fibula
has been broken by the violence of the
muscular activity.

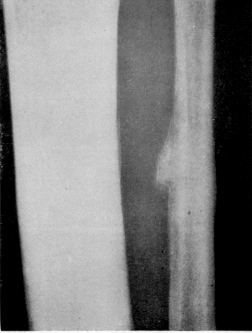

FIG. II.22

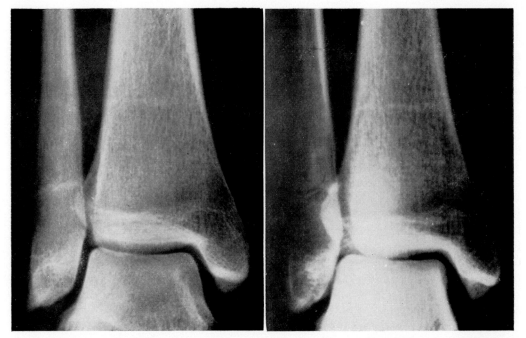

FIG. II.23   FIG. II.24

This athlete has a fracture clearly visible in the radiograph only one week after the onset of symptoms and it is very low down the fibula. There is little disturbance around the fracture, which healed quickly. Figure II.24 shows the appearance two weeks later. This fracture was 3·5 cm from the tip of the lateral malleolus.

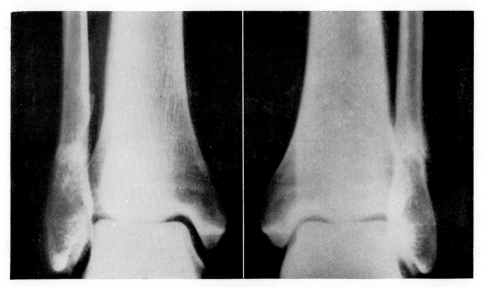

FIG. II.25   FIG. II.26

The disaster that can occur when an athlete takes treatment into his own hands is shown in the radiographs in Figures II.25 and II.26. One ankle having become painful, the athlete decided that he would continue with his training and get rid of the pain by running it off, with the result that the opposite fibula developed a stress fracture. The upward and medial direction of the fracture line is very nicely shown in both figures.

DISCUSSION

It has been shown earlier that the fibula is a non-weight-bearing bone and acts as a strut for muscle origins. It is a very weak strut because it has been shown that simple muscle contraction produces visible movement of the fibula in radiographs (Figs. I.24 and I.25). Thus in the athlete, knowing that the muscle contraction is all-important in producing this stress fracture, activity that exacerbates this unduly can be the cause of the fracture. In particular hard surfaces to which the athlete is unused are dangerous in this respect as is a sudden change from a soft, thick-soled running shoe to a thin-soled plimsoll, which gives less cushioning to each footfall.

In any particular form of sport the circumstances of training, the ground on which it is done and any change in sporting method will all help to establish the full under-standing of the cause of this stress fracture. One other very important consideration is the general physique, fitness and state of training of the athlete or young adult who has undertaken some special activity that is unusual—but not abnormal—because if he attempts to build up muscle power and stamina too quickly he may not allow enough time for the strength of the bone to increase *pari passu* with the strength of the muscles. This is often the case in service recruits. Figures II.27 to II.30 show the radiographs of a sailor in whom this fracture occurred. The radiological development and progress of the fracture is shown with great clarity.

Often an athlete may be stubborn about seeking proper treatment. He may have an important event coming up. He may hope to run off the pain, and in this attitude he may be encouraged by an unwise trainer or other non-medical adviser. It may be suggested that he tries fringe methods such as unskilled massage, horse balm, certain electrical treatments and, most unfortunate of all, hydrocortisone injections with a local anaesthetic. All these treatments are fraught with danger, especially the last method because the freedom from pain for a short while will encourage the athlete to believe that there is nothing seriously wrong. Bilateral stress fractures are an ever-constant hazard as is another stress fracture at a different site. This is more to be expected than as a cause for surprise: if one bone cannot withstand the normal stresses put upon it by the muscles then it is as likely as not that the opposite, or another, bone will also succumb. A stress fracture indicates that the normal strength of any bone has reached its limit of endurance and as a consequence has broken. The dominance of one leg may have a bearing on this but there is no conclusive proof. Finally, the athlete must be impressed on the necessity of resting sufficiently long to enable the bone to unite before he attempts to strengthen it.

Stress Fractures of the Fibula in Children

In young children stress fractures of the fibula are different to those in athletes or middle-aged adults. This difference becomes less as the child grows older and the skeleton becomes more mature, until eventually the stress fracture is usually the same as the runner's fracture in the lowest third of the fibula. This stress fracture is a little more common in boys than girls, particularly in older children.

It is rare to see a stress fracture before the age of 2. A child aged 2, who had just started to walk, began to limp on one leg. Close examination revealed tenderness in both legs (Figs. II.31 to II.34).

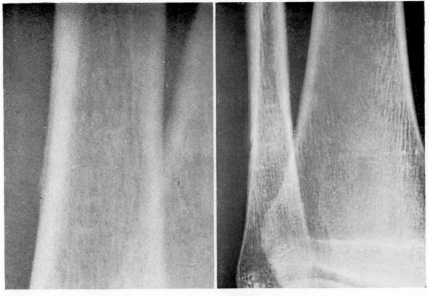

FIG. II.27   FIG. II.28

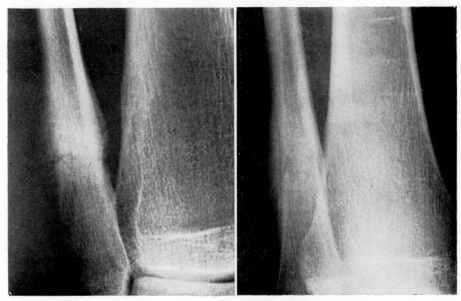

FIG. II.29   FIG. II.30

A sailor aged 20 was perfectly fit until he developed spontaneous pain and swelling on the outer side of his right ankle with no history of injury. He was admitted to a naval hospital where it was found that there was redness and swelling over the lower fibula; the diagnosis of osteomyelitis was considered but a full blood count and other investigations were normal. The radiographs showed an excellent sequence of the developing stress fracture. In Figure II.27 the very early periosteal new bone with the crack just showing in the outer fibula can be seen in an enlarged radiograph but it was only 12 days later that the normal radiograph showed the fracture clearly (Fig. II.28). In a further five weeks the fracture showed a mass of callus across and all round the lower fibula shaft (Fig. II.29) and at three months the fracture was well healed but the crack in the cortex can still be seen (Fig. II.30). There has been no displacement, probably because the sailor concerned was admitted to hospital for investigation and therefore rested it very adequately.

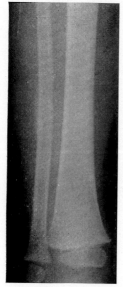 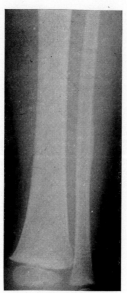 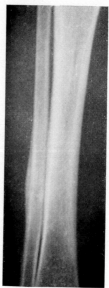 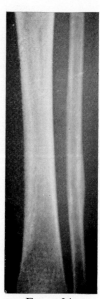

FIG. II.31   FIG. II.32   FIG. II.33   FIG. II.34

The anteroposterior radiographs of a girl aged 2, who had only just started to walk and who had limped on one side, are shown in Figures II.31 and II.32. The parents were unable to tell on which side was the limp; it had been present for no more than one week. The diagnosis was not made at first and full investigation was done with normal results. The second radiographs, shown in Figures II.33 and II.34, are four weeks later and they show the healing of the stress fractures of the middle third of both fibulae.

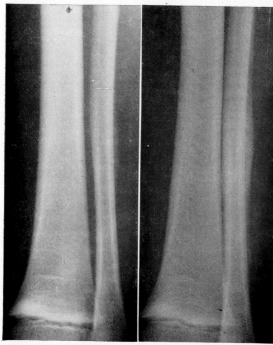

FIG. II.35   FIG. II.36

FIG. II.35   FIG. II.36

Figure II.35 shows the initial radiograph of a girl aged 3½ who was thought by the parents perhaps to have hurt her leg 10 days before. This history is so often the case in a child at this age. Three days after this trivial episode the child complained of pain in the leg. It had begun to improve by the time of the examination when the only finding was a slight tenderness in the lower left fibula. The diagnosis was made on clinical grounds and confirmed by the radiograph. Ten days later the fracture had soundly healed (Fig. II.36).

SYMPTOMS AND SIGNS

The child is brought for advice because of pain, a limp or even general malaise and listlessness. There may be a history of a fever, particularly in the very young, caused by the fracture haematoma. Often there has been some trivial injury which has drawn attention to the pain. The younger the child the more difficulty there is in finding out on which side the limp was, since it is as likely as not to have disappeared at the time of examination; the progress of a stress fracture in a child being so much faster than in the adult. This difficulty is enhanced by a child having bilateral stress fractures, which are not uncommon.

There will be full movement of the ankle and knee but standing on tiptoe will be painful. Palpation of the calf will find a very definite area of tenderness, more on the lateral than medial aspect and most severe over the centre of the shaft of the fibula; in the older child the tenderness is in the lowest third of the fibula, as in the athlete. No swelling will be felt on the fibula nor will there be any very obvious swelling of the leg or ankle as a whole. There will be no obvious wasting.

RADIOLOGY

Within a few days of the start of symptoms in the child the stress fracture is seen radiologically. In the very young, the fracture is longitudinal along the shaft of the fibula. As the child grows older the fracture occurs in the lower fibula. At first there is new bone formation which appears to be under the periosteum. It may be extremely faint, as in Figures II.35 and II.36, which shows the development of the typical callus in a young child. The whole width of the shaft of the fibula may be involved, as shown in Figures II.37 and II.38. The older child, after the lower fibula epiphysis has united, develops the typical runner's fracture (Figs. II.39 and II.40). Figures II.41 and II.42 are the radiographs of a boy of $17\frac{1}{2}$ who had a stress fracture in the lower third of the left fibula the year before and who developed pain in the same leg which he attempted to run off. He was seized with an acute and sudden pain in the calf of the opposite right leg, having run four and a half miles. The right fibula had a comminuted stress fracture which must have been present as a partial fracture but the symptoms were hidden by those of the stress fracture high up in the left fibula.

The bone of a young child is more malleable than that of the adolescent. It may even, without showing a fracture line, develop slight angulation with a stress fracture. Figures II.43 and II.44 are the radiographs of a boy of 7 who was brought to hospital with a history of ten days pain in the leg but which had already stopped by the time the radiographs were taken. Despite the slight angulation the symptoms were brief.

The progress of an interesting fracture in a boy of 8 is shown in Figures II.45 and II.46. He was radiographed for a painful limp which had been present for one week and which had started after skating. In the first radiograph (Fig. II.45) the crack can be seen quite clearly going through the outer cortex of the fibula and running for some distance up the shaft of the fibula. In the later radiograph at six weeks (Fig. II.46) there is a considerable change: the fracture has become complete, involving the medial cortex, and the longitudinal crack is shown by the long slim line of new bone formation on the outer side of the fibula. Here again there has been very slight deformity, but healing is now almost complete and all symptoms had stopped. It is doubtful if the

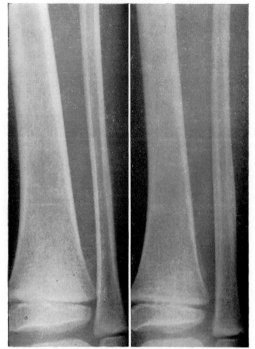

FIG. II.37   FIG. II.38

FIG. II.37   FIG. II.38

The radiograph of a boy aged 5 is shown in Figure II.37. It shows what was correctly diagnosed as a stress fracture but some anxiety existed as to whether a sarcoma could cause this appearance. In the first radiograph the slight haze of new bone could arouse suspicion; but after a short interval the second radiograph (Fig. II.38) dispelled all doubt.

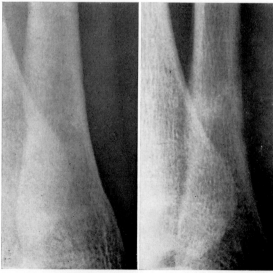

FIG. II.39   FIG. II.40

FIG. II.39   FIG. II.40

The first radiograph of a boy of 16, who was an athlete, is shown in Figure II.39. He had recently changed his training from soft ground to hard and in a little while developed pain in the outer side of the left leg just above the ankle. The early and minute crack in the outer cortex of the lowest third of the fibula can just be seen; three to four weeks later the fracture was healing well in the radiograph in Figure II.40.

Fig. II.41   Fig. II.42

The radiographs of a schoolboy aged 17 who has had three stress fractures. Not all stress fractures are entirely straightforward; and this youth had had, the year previously, a stress fracture of the lowest third of the left fibula, of which the healed remains can be seen in Figure II.42. While running he developed pain in the outer side of the left leg which spoilt his form. He continued to train to try and 'run it off'. Three weeks later, having run four and a half miles, he felt a sudden sharp pain in the outer calf (Fig. II.41). He had bilateral stress fractures of the middle thirds of both fibulae; at first the left, being painful, had masked the pain on the right. With obstinacy and endurance the boy continued to run until the weakened area of the shaft of the right fibula gave way completely and splintered. Despite the fibula not being a weight-bearing bone there has been slight compression of the fragments.

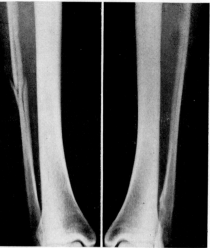

Fig. II.41   Fig. II.42

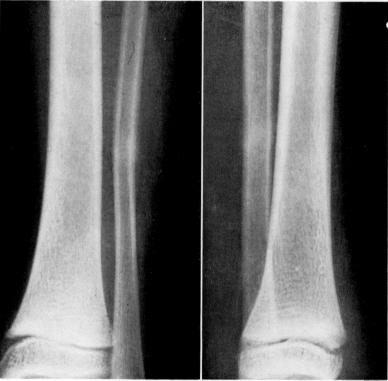

Fig. II.43   Fig. II.44

A boy of 7 had grazed his left leg 10 days before he was seen for the ache which had continued thereafter. The radiographs, when he first attended, showed a typical stress fracture, and one which indicates that the fracture is becoming more localised at this age than it is in the younger child, although still fairly high up in the shaft of the fibula. The anteroposterior view suggests that there has been slight angulation at the site of the fracture. The lateral radiograph shows very clearly the almost horizontal fracture line.

history of skating is important except as an unusual activity to which he was perhaps not accustomed.

DIAGNOSIS

The diagnosis of a stress fracture in a child is not always as easy as it seems it ought to be because the pain is not severe and often the child is not brought early for advice; usually the symptoms are already waning by the time the child is seen. If the onset has by chance been sudden and severe there may be, for the first day or two, little to be seen in the radiographs to confirm the diagnosis. Careful clinical examination, however, will have found the tenderness around the fibula. Listlessness, with a slight irregular fever but no swelling with the tenderness, is usual in the very young; finally, the rapid cessation of symptoms once the child is put to bed is very helpful.

The important differential diagnosis is a neoplasm, and many fibulae have had a biopsy done upon them to exclude this. Sometimes the appearance of callus in the radiograph is highly suggestive of a sarcoma, as in Figure II.47; the biopsy from this boy showed normal new bone formation (Fig. II.48). If the natural history of a stress fracture is understood, the speed of progress by the time arrangements have been made for the child to be admitted to hospital for the biopsy and further radiography will usually exclude a neoplasm. If doubt does still exist, the biopsy should be done.

Infantile cortical hyperostosis, with its new bone formation, will not be difficult to differentiate because a stress fracture is entirely localised to one fibula or occasionally to both. The 'battered baby' syndrome must be considered in the very young child but absence of bruising and other injury should be cause for this diagnosis to be discarded. Pain, tenderness, malaise and fever may suggest osteomyelitis, but observation will show that the fever is slight and irregular and that there is a very rapid improvement with rest in bed. Rickets or scurvy could confuse, but the brevity of the existence of a stress fracture and the rapid radiological changes will be sufficient to establish the correct diagnosis.

TREATMENT

For children the only treatment needed is to stop the excess activity that causes the pain, sometimes with simple supportive bandaging of the lower leg in the older child, as for the athlete. Symptoms soon cease in the younger child but take longer to go in the adolescent, especially if the stress fracture of the fibula is of the type seen in athletes, and this may take four to six weeks to settle.

There is no anxiety that a child with a stress fracture is in any way unhealthy and no general treatment is needed.

There is no way of preventing an active child getting this fracture within the confines of a normal life; but in the athletic adolescent the normal methods of training and the wearing of proper shoes will help, as has been discussed earlier in this chapter.

DISCUSSION

Stress fractures of the fibula occur in the very young to the very elderly; at all ages the aetiology is the same, that is, the muscular pull bending the fibula towards the tibia. It would be surprising if young children did not get this fracture, in the same way that they also get a stress fracture of the tibia. It is not a very common occurrence

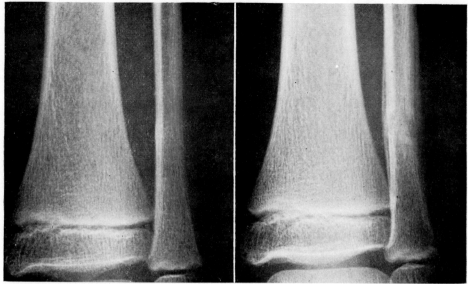

FIG. II.45   FIG. II.46

A boy of 8 had a history of about one week's pain in the outer aspect of his left lower leg. The first anteroposterior radiograph (Fig. II.45) shows the earliest outline of the stress fracture in a child, a crack through the outer cortex extending longitudinally upwards in the shaft of the fibula. Thereafter the change was rapid and six weeks later the extent of the whole lesion can be seen (Fig. II.46). By now all symptoms had stopped.

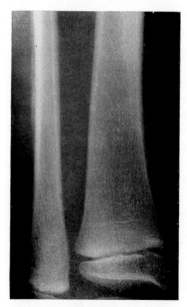
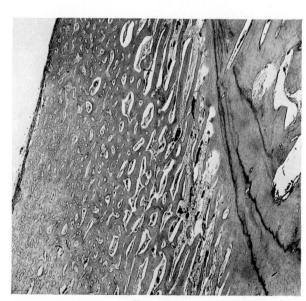

FIG. II.47   FIG. II.48

A boy aged 3 complained of pain in the left leg fairly low down which had been present for some three weeks when he was seen in a clinic. He was admitted forthwith for biopsy with a presumptive diagnosis of a sarcoma (Fig. II.47). At examination slight induration over the lower fibula was found; it was very tender. There was no past history of note except that a fish-hook had caught in his right leg some 10 months previously leaving a very small scar. The child improved while awaiting the biopsy which was done a week after first being seen and this showed healthy normal callus (Fig. II.48).

in children and is not seen as often as the stress fractures in athletes or in the middle-aged adult.

Children who have had a stress fracture develop normally thereafter with no evidence of any systemic disease as a precursor. It should always be borne in mind, however, that if a child develops a stress fracture which does not follow the normal pattern or natural history, then the suspicion that there may be another cause must be investigated.

Stress Fractures of the Fibula in Middle Age

In middle-age a woman is much more vulnerable to a stress fracture of the lowest third of the fibula than is a man. The reasons for this difference are obscure without placing the whole blame on postmenopausal osteoporosis causing a weakening of the bone. It is also just possible that the activity of the women affected may have increased but this is unlikely to be more than a cause in a few patients.

SYMPTOMS AND SIGNS

The symptoms are usually typical. Pain starts in the ankle and gradually gets worse. It is felt on the outer side and it may radiate to the outer border of the foot; it is worse after activity, in the evening and at rest at night. The patient will often recall some trivial episode of unusual activity that started, or drew attention to, the symptoms (Fig. II.49 and II.50). Sometimes the pain comes on rapidly over a few days although usually the history is of pain slowly increasing until it is bad enough to cause the patient to seek attention (Figs. II.51 to II.53); the history of this patient draws attention to the common finding of some unusual, but not abnormal, episode of activity.

Figure II.54 shows the radiograph of a woman of 67 who had rheumatoid arthritis but who had never been treated with steroids. The stress fracture is quite typical and the radiograph does not suggest any marked osteoporosis.

Patients may have a history of some other condition causing deformity, such as arthritis (Fig. II.55 and II.56) or Paget's disease. Although the latter may predispose to stress fractures in the affected bone, it may also cause stress fractures by reason of the altered weight-bearing or posture (Figs. II.57 to II.59).

A history of any gastrointestinal complaint, and especially of a gastrectomy or a similar operation, is important because malabsorption can predispose to osteoporosis, which may not be apparent clinically but which may be sufficient to precipitate a stress fracture.

The clinical examination will usually show a healthy patient, most often a woman, but rarely with some other systemic disease such as rheumatoid arthritis, Paget's disease or osteoporosis. Abdominal scars may indicate a gastrectomy; deformities of the limbs should be noted. Locally the ankle will be swollen but no swelling on the lower fibula itself can be discerned because of the general oedema. This is different from the young patient or athlete in whom such local swelling can sometimes be seen. Often there is slight swelling of the opposite ankle and, because of the rather vague nature of the pain, the normally acutely tender spot about 5 cm from the tip of the lateral malleolus may not be found. The swelling of the fibula can be palpated unless there is very severe swelling of the ankle as a whole. The ankle itself may have some general tenderness and the foot may be painful because the patient has walked

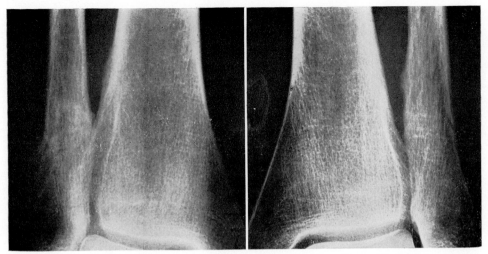

FIG. II.49   FIG. II.50

A woman at the age of 51 developed pain in the right ankle on its outer side two weeks before being seen. The pain had come on suddenly. The radiograph (Fig. II.49) shows a typical stress fracture of the right fibula in its lowest third. It is interesting that two years later she attended with the same condition (Fig. II.50) with a history that she had noticed the pain for one week after knocking the ankle against a chair. The two stress fractures are almost identical. She was treated in the usual adhesive strapping and was perfectly fit within eight weeks.

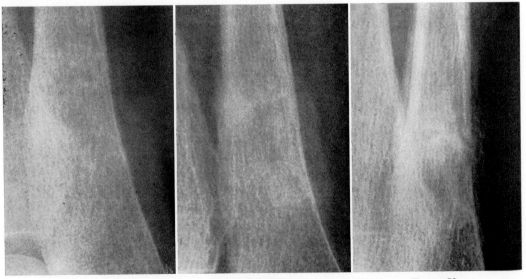

FIG. II.51   FIG. II.52   FIG. II.53

A woman of 58 had had a pain in the right fibula for six weeks. Before this she was leading a normal life but had recently been to stay with a sister who lived beside an unmade road in the country. Gradually she had noticed pain and swelling, both of which were worse at night. The radiograph in Figure II.51 shows a typical stress fracture of the lowest third of the fibula which is developing slowly. The slight haze of new bone can be seen on the lateral cortex of the fibula and also in two places, one above the other, across the bone itself. The further development of the callus in these two areas is well shown in Figure II.52, which was taken ten days later, but it was only after a further five weeks that the actual fracture in the outer cortex of the fibula was visible in the radiograph shown in Figure II.53.

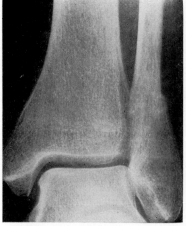

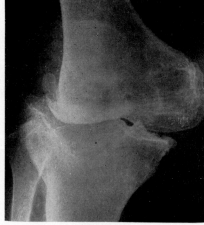

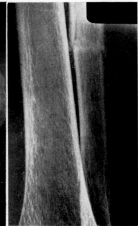

FIG. II.54   FIG. II.55   FIG. II.56

A woman of 67 had rheumatoid arthritis and was diagnosed clinically as suffering from a stress fracture of the lower fibula. The patient was not on steroids. The radiographs were seen and the diagnosis was confirmed but at that time the diagnosis of a stress fracture of the tibia, which can just be seen in the radiographs, was not made (see Chapter IV). The patient recovered with rest.

A deformity will predispose to a stress fracture. An elderly lady of 82 developed a stress fracture at the junction of the middle and lower thirds of the shaft of the fibula. The radiograph shows a severe deformity of the knee (Fig. II.55). The deformity, not only predisposing to a stress fracture, has produced abnormal stress with an unusual stress fracture as shown in the radiograph (Fig. II.56).

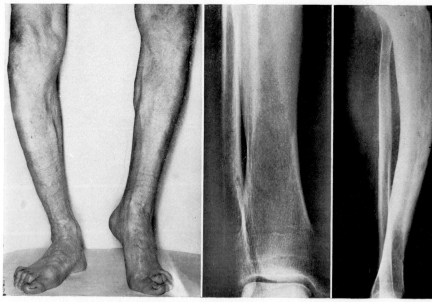

FIG. II.57   FIG. II.58   FIG. II.59

Figure II.57 shows the appearance of the legs of a man of 70 who had severe Paget's disease. There is much bowing of the right lower leg. He had complained of pain in the right ankle; there was not much swelling but he was tender in the usual position just at, and above, the lateral malleolus. The anteroposterior radiograph (Fig. II.58) shows that there is a stress fracture in the lowest third of the right fibula but that the fracture line is running from the medial side upwards and laterally, because of the altered direction of stress from the deformity which is shown in Figure II.59.

awkwardly in trying to alleviate the pain. The swelling of the fibula, at first soft, soon becomes hard as callus is formed. Pressure on the shaft of the fibula above the fracture may cause pain at the site of the stress fracture. Straining the ankle in a manner to pull or push the lateral malleolus may also cause pain but these tests are far less reliable than the actual point of tenderness that is always present at the site of the stress fracture. In the very old patient the tibia can also have a stress fracture, with more swelling, more pain and much more difficulty in walking, but these double stress fractures are dealt with in Chapter IV.

Sometimes stress fractures of the fibula are bilateral but very rarely are they bilateral at the same time. Normally there is an interval of months or years, as is shown in Figures II.49 and II.50 and also in Figures II.60 to II.63.

RADIOLOGY

In the middle-aged it is more common to find the early radiological changes of a stress fracture of the lower fibula when the patient is first seen, but by no means always so. This is because the stress fracture has already existed for several weeks by the time the patient seeks advice or is referred for radiography. The symptoms are most often gradual in their development and are rarely so sudden or acute that the patient has to be seen at once.

Figures II.60 to II.63 do, however, show an extremely early stress fracture in a patient who had been warned that the opposite ankle might develop a stress fracture after the original lesion. The original fracture in the left ankle is shown in Figures II.60 and II.61. The very small crack of the second fracture in the posterolateral aspect of the lower right fibula was shown at two days after the onset of the symptoms by careful radiological positioning when the fracture was not seen in the normal anteroposterior or lateral views. Five weeks later the fracture was obvious (Fig. II.63) and the lateral view shows a very similar pattern to that of the opposite ankle (Figs. II.60 and II.61). It is interesting that in the interval of five weeks between the radiographs in Figures II.62 and II.63 the fracture developed to involve the whole of the fibula despite treatment and has even become displaced slightly, though less than the previous fracture on the opposite side.

Generally the fracture line runs upwards and medially from the posterolateral cortex in the same way as it does in the athlete. Most fractures become complete unless caught very early and unless the ankle has been immobilised in plaster of Paris. Serial radiography will show the complete fracture some weeks after the onset of symptoms; the fracture line may be transverse from the oblique crack in the outer cortex across the shaft (Figs. II.64 and II.65) or has the appearance of a double spiral in one radiograph but which is shown to be a simple fracture in other views (Figs. II.66 and II.67).

Without serial radiographs it might often be thought that the fracture was not complete because the symptoms soon stop and final radiographs do not seem necessary. In Figures II.68 to II.70 are shown the radiographs of the stress fracture in a man; the original radiograph showed a very small haze of callus on the outer side of the lower fibula; an oblique view one week later showed an increase in the callus. Two weeks later, that is three weeks after symptoms had started, the callus has increased and a haze of new bone formation can be seen right across the shaft of the lower fibula. If this radiograph had not been taken (for which there was no clinical necessity) it might have been thought that the fracture was only through part of the bone.

D

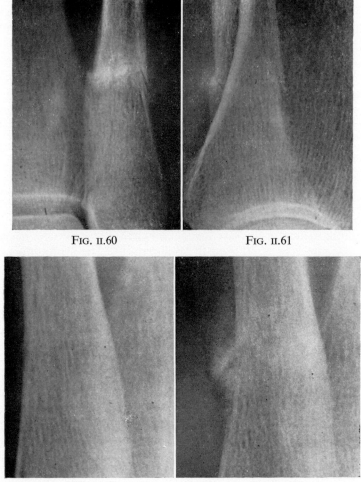

FIG. II.60   FIG. II.61

FIG. II.62   FIG. II.63

A woman of 57 went on holiday and did more than her usual amount of walking both in town and country. She developed pain and swelling in the left ankle, mostly on the outer side; this later became acute and when she presented some months after the onset of symptoms the fracture was clearly seen in the radiographs and was already uniting (Figs. II.60 and II.61). It is worth noting that the fracture line runs upwards and inwards (or proximally and medially) from the outer cortex of the fibula to extend in an irregular manner across the shaft. In the lateral view the fracture line can be seen running upwards at the back of the fibula where it has involved the posterolateral cortex. There is ample callus around the fracture but firm union was not present. Simple supportive bandaging was sufficient to cure this patient's symptoms, and she was warned that occasionally this fracture could affect both sides. Some ten weeks later she returned with a history of starting pain only two days previously in the opposite right ankle. Radiographs were taken with great care and many views were done, and one of the oblique projections showed a very small crack in the lateral cortex of the right fibula above the malleolus (Fig. II.62). The patient was given firm support and, as can be seen from the radiograph taken five weeks later (Fig. II.63), the fracture did not become so severe in its appearance as the previous fracture on the left side which had first been treated a long time after onset. The fracture has probably involved the whole cortex but it has certainly not displaced itself to any extent. It is also important to note that the fracture line can be seen passing down through the callus, which indicates that movement is still occurring at the fracture site. If this is to be avoided, absolute immobilisation in a plaster cast has to be used but it is usually not necessary in ordinary patients although an athlete might be an exception.

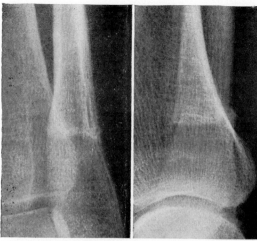 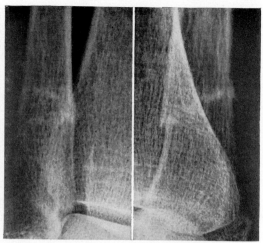

FIG. II.64   FIG. II.65   FIG. II.66   FIG. II.67

A middle-aged woman had injured her chest in an accident six weeks before being seen but did not injure her ankle. Three weeks later the ankle began to hurt and after a further two weeks the radiographs showed a typical stress fracture but with slight compression of the fragments. She was treated in elastic adhesive bandages.

A woman of 68 years developed sudden pain in the lateral side of the right ankle while walking downstairs some weeks before the radiograph was taken. Figure II.66 shows the line of the fracture encircling the lower fibula, and in the lateral view (Fig. II.67) it can be seen that the line is not so much callus formation as a slight compression of the fragments. Very often a sudden pain indicates that the stress fracture has abruptly become complete.

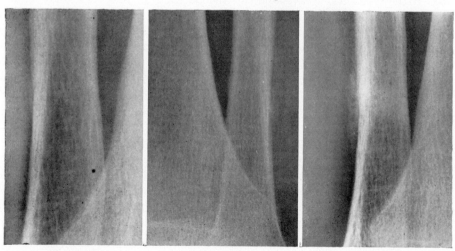

FIG. II.68   FIG. II.69   FIG. II.70

A man of 61 felt a sudden pain just above the outer side of his right ankle while walking. He was seen the next day and found to have a tender swelling above the lateral malleolus. The radiograph showed slight periosteal callus just above the right lateral malleolus, only seen in the oblique view (Fig. II.68). Figure II.69 is a radiograph of the same ankle one week later and the callus is now a little bit more abundant. Two weeks later (Fig. II.70) the callus was clearly seen and also the haze of new bone, or internal callus, going across the shaft of the lower fibula. He was treated by strapping and he was free of symptoms in just over six weeks.

Aids to radiography are not needed in this age group. Careful marking of the site of the stress fracture so that the radiographer may obtain good pictures centred on the lesion is all that is necessary. This is important, as is the request for at least one oblique view to show the posterolateral aspect of the fibula particularly in the early stages of the condition.

DIAGNOSIS

The diagnosis of stress fractures of the lower fibula in middle age is made on clinical grounds. The history of increasing pain after exercise, then with exercise, aching in the evening and finally severe pain both with exercise and at rest is typical; when the tender area on the lower fibula is found and the local swelling felt at that site there should be no doubt as to the cause.

To differentiate from other conditions in this age group is not arduous because the history and clinical signs are easy to interpret with the exception of the simultaneous stress fractures of the tibia and fibula, or the compression stress fracture of the lower tibia. However, any general condition that might cause pain in the ankle, such as rheumatoid arthritis or osteoarthritis, should be excluded, as should intermittent claudication from vascular disease. Osteoporosis may precipitate a stress fracture.

Particular local conditions may confuse, such as varicose veins, especially with a small superficial thrombosis; a tenosynovitis near the lateral malleolus although not common can occur; finally the lack of signs of acute inflammation will exclude infection.

TREATMENT

As in the athlete, the best treatment is to support the ankle in elastic adhesive strapping. If the condition is explained to the patients so that they understand that they will still get a little pain doing household duties or other activities, they will be prepared to accept it. Furthermore, they can all be assured that the pain will go in about four weeks, or at the most six, and if they are able to rest or cut down their activities the pain will be eased even more. Very rarely is the pain sufficient to make it necessary to put the patient into a below-knee plaster cast on which he may walk. After the strapping is removed physiotherapy may be needed in this group of patients, partly because they are liable to swelling of the ankles anyway, for which Faradism under pressure may be indicated, and also to restore the tone of the intrinsic muscles of the foot and of the calf and to ensure that the ankle regains its former mobility.

To try and prevent stress fractures in all middle-aged women by making them use thick-soled rubber shoes, cutting down their excursions or shopping sprees and otherwise interfering with their daily life would be insufferable; but once a stress fracture has occurred the particular incident that caused it can be drawn to the patient's attention and, with advice on footwear, measures against a second stress fracture may be of value. There is no doubt that a thick and soft-soled shoe will cushion the foot against excessive contraction of the calf muscles for the unaccustomed activity.

DISCUSSION

The stress fracture of the lower fibula that occurs in middle age is usually seen in women. Osteoporosis may be a factor in this. The fracture is caused by the bending of the fibula from the muscle pull that has been described earlier in this chapter, and which occurs in running or walking. The apparent compression that is seen in the complete fracture is secondary and is occasioned by the continued pull of the muscles with walking or other activity; the top of the fibula is not firmly fixed so it is reasonable to expect that it could be pulled down and compressed at the fracture site.

The common site of the start of the fracture, the posterolateral cortex just above the malleolus, is where the bend in the fibula is the greatest with normal activity and where the pull, or distraction, on the outer cortex is most concentrated. A small crack starts, then progresses upwards and inwards through the lateral cortex. Once this is broken through, the weakened bone can then break completely.

This stress fracture of the fibula is often seen in everyday clinical practice. It is now so well known that patients should be diagnosed and treated by their general practitioner without a visit to hospital or resource to radiography. The satisfactory progress of the patient over a few weeks confirms the diagnosis.

There is another form of stress fracture of the fibula which occurs in the elderly; this is the simultaneous stress fracture of the fibula and the tibia which is seen in old people who are active and sometimes healthy, sometimes with clinical osteoporosis. It is of great interest because it is a compression stress fracture of the lower ends of both the tibia and of the fibula with the line of the fracture running across the two bones and situated either above the ankle or just below the knee. These simultaneous stress fractures of the tibia and fibula are described in Chapter Four.

CHAPTER THREE

STRESS FRACTURES OF THE TIBIA

Introduction

The tibia is the most interesting bone in which to study stress fractures because it shows such a variety of reactions to stress. Basically the cross section of the tibia is triangular, which is an unusual shape for a bone that has to take very high strains both from the weight passing through the bone as well as very intense muscular stresses imposed upon it in such actions as running or jumping; it is not surprising, therefore, that the tibia sustains many different stress fractures.

Both compression and distraction stress fractures occur in the tibia and they are easily divisible into various clinical and radiological groups. Figures III.1 to III.5 show radiological examples of each type and each illustration is typical of the age, activity and clinical findings of the patient concerned.

The child develops a compression stress fracture of the upper tibia (Fig. III.1) at which site the elderly person also develops a similar stress fracture but not so commonly as in the lowest part of the tibia (Fig. III.4); the latter are often associated with a stress fracture of the fibula at the same level. These are described separately in Chapter Four.

Distraction stress fractures can be divided into oblique (Fig. III.2), longitudinal (Fig. III.3) and transverse (Fig. III.5) and are easily distinguished radiologically but much less easy to distinguish clinically. However, any stress fracture at the middle of the tibial shaft must be considered to be transverse until proved otherwise as it is particularly dangerous because of the ease with which a complete and displaced fracture may occur.

There is a difference in the pattern of the fracture according to the age and activity of the patient, but again this is not so clear-cut in the distraction as in the compression stress fracture. It must be emphasised that although stress fractures in general may be either compression or distraction, the further subdivision of such fractures in the tibia does not necessarily hold true for other bones. Thus the compression fracture of the calcaneus is common in the young or middle-aged adult, as is the distraction stress fracture of the tibia. Compression stress fractures of the femoral neck also occur in young adults as well as in the elderly, and in each group the distraction stress fracture may also occur. Usually the compression stress fracture is much less liable to lead to disability and heals well although those in the femoral neck may be exceptions to this.

The medial malleolus, the tibial tubercle and the tibial plateau have stress fractures peculiar to themselves.

In the tibia compression and distraction stress fractures occur equally. Of the former half are in children and half in elderly adults; of the latter most are oblique to cause shin soreness. About one in ten are longitudinal and about one in 20 are transverse;

46

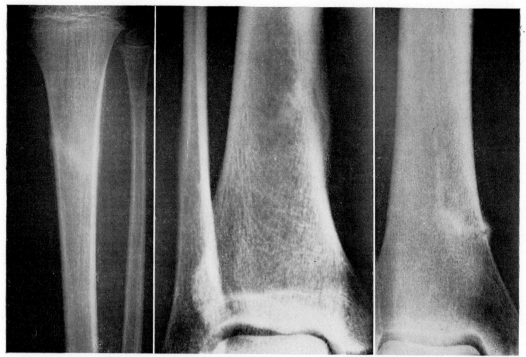

FIG. III.1   FIG. III.2   FIG. III.3

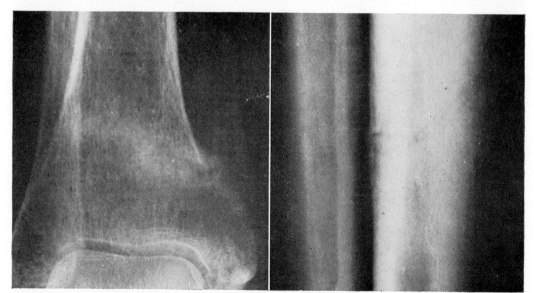

FIG. III.4   FIG. III.5

The radiographs of the five important varieties of stress fracture of the tibia are shown here. In Figure III.1 is the radiograph of a compression stress fracture in a child of 5. Figure III.2 shows the oblique stress fracture in the radiograph of an athlete aged 21 who complained of shin soreness. Figure III.3 is the radiograph of a middle-aged woman with a longitudinal stress fracture that is seen running up the shaft from the crack in the cortex at the lowest third of the tibia. Figure III.4 shows a compression stress fracture in the radiograph of a woman of 54. Finally, Figure III.5 shows the transverse stress fracture in the centre of the tibial shaft in the radiograph of an international footballer.

although the latter are one of the more rare stress fractures they can cause severe disability if not diagnosed and treated correctly.

Stress Fractures of the Tibia in Children

Compression stress fractures are seen in children from infancy until the skeletal maturity of the tibia, which occurs at about the age of 16 years. There is also a much rarer type of longitudinal stress fracture which accounts for only about one in ten of these stress fractures seen in children. When the child has become physically mature the oblique type of tibial stress fracture takes the place of the compression stress fracture.

The compression stress fracture in children is never lower than at the junction of the middle and uppermost third of the tibia. The change in the way the tibia reacts to stress relates not to the actual age of the child but to the muscular development, strength and the cessation of rapid growth in the leg and the alteration of the bone itself from the malleable growing bone to the more rigid structure of the adult. This again emphasises that stress fractures are not caused by a heavy footfall but by strong repeated muscular contractions stressing the bone; according to the stress and the age of the bone one or another form of stress fracture occurs.

In children, boys are affected more often than girls but the difference is not great, being approximately three boys to two girls, and the compression stress fractures are remarkably similar whatever the sex or age. Figures III.6 to III.8 show the radiographs of a girl of 17 months who had started to walk with a stiff right leg two weeks previously and who had no history of injury. If that appearance is compared to Figures III.9 and III.10, which are the radiographs of a boy of 16 who was a cross-country runner, it will be seen that the two fractures are alike yet the older boy had a typical history of shin soreness, with pain coming on at first after and then during exercise; also he had been training on roads. Despite this, but perhaps because the upper tibial epiphysis is still just visible, he developed a compression stress fracture, and not the oblique stress fracture common to runners which also can occur at this level in the tibia.

Symptoms and Signs

The onset of symptoms in the child occurs in much the same way as stress fractures in general, but the younger the child the faster the progress, so that in most tibial stress fractures the disability has probably been apparent for not much more than two or three weeks; the radiological changes follow with equal rapidity. Very often by the time the child has been brought for medical advice the radiograph may show that the fracture is healing. The older the child, the longer is the course, until at about the age of 16 it may take the same time for a compression stress fracture to recover as in the adult with shin soreness caused by the oblique stress fracture through the tibial cortex.

Examination in the early days of a stress fracture in a young child will show a tender, painful, red swelling just below the knee, the most acutely tender area being medially on the subcutaneous part of the tibia or on its posteromedial edge. There will be no enlarged glands and, although there may be slight malaise and fever in the early stages, often by the time the child is seen not only is there no malaise but the redness and tenderness has improved. The swelling does not affect the knee, in which there is no fluid. Movement of the knee and ankle is full but the child walks with a limp.

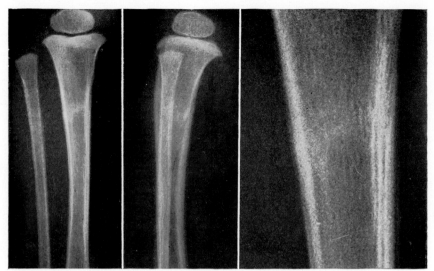

FIG. III.6   FIG. III.7   FIG. III.8

A child aged 17 months was seen with a short history of walking stiff-legged on the right side, and the parents thought that the leg was thinner than the left. There was no history of injury. On enquiry it was elicited that two weeks before being seen the child had not wanted to put her foot down but later had walked in the fashion described. Radiologically there is a compression stress fracture in the uppermost third of the tibia which has involved more the lateral and posterior part of the bone although the internal callus can be seen very clearly, particularly in Figure III.8, which is an enlargement of Figure III.6.

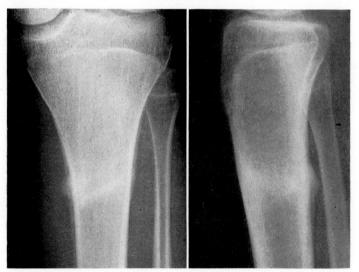

FIG. III.9   FIG. III.10

An athletic boy of 16 who did a lot of cross-country running said that he first noticed pain when he knocked his leg against a chair five weeks before being seen. About a week later he was still able to run but 'something went' while he was road-running. When seen he had a hot, tender swelling in the upper and medial part of the left shin. The radiographs show the compression stress fracture and also that the periosteum has not only been elevated from the bone medially, laterally and posteriorly, but also appears to have ruptured so that some callus is forming outside the line of the periosteal elevation. It may well have been this occurrence that caused the feeling of 'something going' in his leg whilst running.

RADIOLOGY

A fully developed stress fracture is shown in Figures III.11 and III.12, which are the radiographs of a boy aged 8 who had had Köhler's disease of the navicular bone on the same side; having recovered from that he developed pain in the shin. Rest in bed or in a splint, or even avoiding weight-bearing on crutches is always a potential cause of a stress fracture at all ages.

In some children the very earliest radiological sign is a slight haze of callus in the shaft of the tibia. Figures III.13 and III.14 show the upper tibiae of a girl of 12. Having been correctly diagnosed as a stress fracture of the right tibia she was put into plaster for seven weeks—which was much too long—and when it was removed the fracture of the opposite tibia was apparent. Both tibiae show well the internal callus that is formed by a compression stress fracture. The haze across the shaft of the bone, whether it shows in the anteroposterior or lateral view, is only internal callus and often there is no break in the cortex of the tibia. Sometimes at a later stage not only does the cortex fracture but the periosteum may be elevated over a considerable distance by new bone forming in a subperiosteal haematoma. This is shown well in Figures III.15 to III.17. Rarely the periosteum itself is ruptured to allow the extrusion of callus into the surrounding tissues (Figs. III.9 and III.10).

Longitudinal Stress Fracture of the Tibia in Children

The rare longitudinal stress fracture in a child is to be recognised by a very faint periosteal shadow; this is long and thin and is well shown in the radiographs of a girl of $2\frac{1}{2}$ with pain in the right leg. The first radiograph was normal (Fig. III.18) but ten days later (Fig. III.19) there was a line of periosteal new bone down most of the lateral cortex of the tibia. Two months later all that is seen is thickening of the tibial shaft as a whole but mostly on the lateral cortex (Fig. III.20).

Another radiological example is shown in Figures III.21 and III.22. When the stress fracture was first diagnosed it appeared to show only at the posterior cortex (Fig. III.21) but five weeks later the fracture could be seen passing up and down the shaft (Fig. III.22).

In any radiograph the state of the epiphyseal plate is to be noted because if it is still widely open it will suggest the type of fracture to be expected. When the upper tibial epiphysis is united then the stress fracture will be of an adult type.

DIAGNOSIS

This is not difficult. The symptoms of pain with no injury, or an almost painless limp, the local swelling and tenderness, and the radiological changes that are usually early will establish the diagnosis provided this occurrence of such a stress fracture of the tibia is well understood.

TREATMENT

Most children need no treatment other than reassurance and advice on which activities they should not undertake. So often the young child has healed his fracture by the time he is brought for attention. The older child may be put off games and told not to romp or rush about too much, and the more mature adolescent may have to be put off sport and have the leg supported in elastic adhesive strapping for a week or two but usually it is also reasonably quick to unite. It is very rare that the

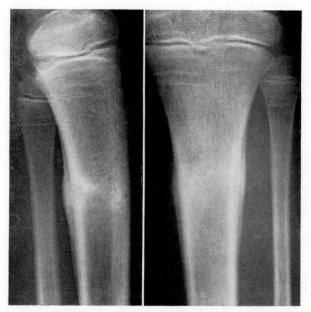

FIG. III.11   FIG. III.12

This boy of 8 shows the classical radiological appearance of a compression stress fracture in a child. There is a haze of bone running across the shaft with subperiosteal new bone, particularly posteriorly and also on each side of the tibia, but little or none in front. It is interesting that he had had Köhler's disease of the left navicular bone, from which symptoms had started two years previously, but he had been free of pain in the foot for two months before he got pain in the tibia. The rapidity of the symptoms in the child makes it easy to become suspicious of a stress fracture, particularly when there is no history of injury or other symptoms.

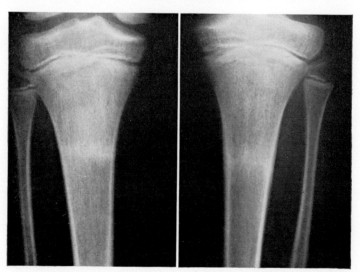

FIG. III.13   FIG.III.14

A girl of 12 developed pain in the right upper tibia. She was diagnosed as a stress fracture and was treated in plaster for seven weeks. At the end of that time she had pain in the opposite tibia and it is clear that both tibial radiographs show stress fractures. In a poor-quality radiograph the fracture might easily be overlooked.

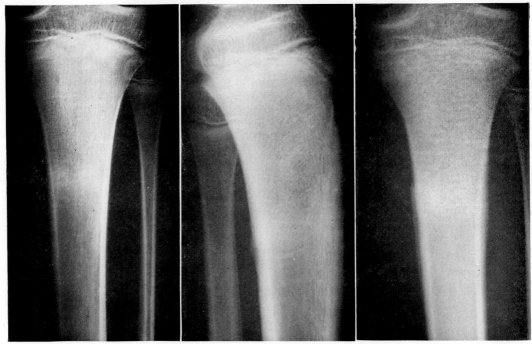

FIG. III.15   FIG. III.16   FIG. III.17

A girl aged 9 complained of pain in the upper left shin for two to three months. There was no history of injury. When first seen there was a slight haze of internal callus in the radiograph of the left tibia (Fig. III.15). There was a small break in the cortex posteriorly (Fig. III.16), and a month later the typical appearance of a compression stress fracture was seen (Fig. III.17).

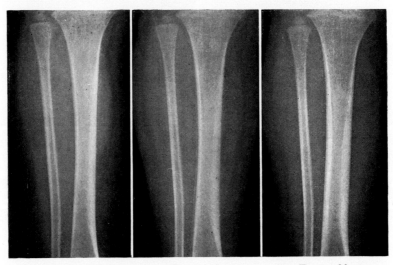

FIG. III.18   FIG. III.19   FIG. III.20

A girl of $2\frac{1}{2}$ years was brought to hospital with pain and tenderness in the lower part of her right leg. The first radiograph appeared to be normal (Fig. III.18) but ten days later (Fig. III.19) there was a faint periosteal shadow down the lateral cortex of the tibia. After a further two months there is little to be seen except general thickening of the tibia on its lateral cortex (Fig. III.20). Investigations and follow-up disproved that she had infantile cortical hyperostosis or that she had the 'battered baby' syndrome. This is one of the rare longitudinal stress fractures of the tibia in a child.

symptoms are so severe that an above-knee plaster cast is needed on which the child may walk provided it does not hurt. A below-knee walking plaster or a cylinder allows full weight to pass through the stress fracture, and pain continues. It is easier, if there is much pain, to put the child non-weight-bearing on crutches for a few days when the symptoms will have improved greatly and walking will be resumed very quickly.

There is no evidence that children who get this condition are in any way osteo-porotic or suffering from malnutrition or any other generalised disease.

DISCUSSION

The vagueness of the symptoms, particularly in a young child seen late, may cause slight difficulty in diagnosis, especially as to which bone is affected. A stress fracture can occur in the fibula with very much the same history; Figure III.23 shows the radio-graph of a boy aged $2\frac{1}{2}$ who had a stress fracture of the right fibula. Eight months later he returned with more pain in the leg and another radiograph was normal; he continued to limp and a further radiograph one month later showed the stress fracture in his tibia (Fig. III.24).

Osteochondritis of the tibial tubercle has localised tenderness so that it is easily distinguished from the stress fracture of the upper tibia.

The various systemic diseases can be discounted where the general health of the child is good and there is otherwise complete fitness on examination. Also it is unlikely that disease of the knee will confuse since a stress fracture allows free movement when not weight-bearing and causes no fluid in the joint. Acute osteomyelitis is distinguished by the high fever, malaise and shorter history; a Brodie's abscess, on the other hand, can mislead but is recognisable radiologically.

A sarcoma may cause an appearance not very different from a stress fracture. Figure III.25 shows, radiologically, an osteogenic sarcoma at the junction of the middle and uppermost thirds of the right tibia which is not all that different from the stress fracture adjacent to it shown in the radiograph in Figure III.26. If there is any doubt about the diagnosis the child should be admitted and a biopsy done; but a radiograph taken after the child has had the usual tests often will confirm the diagnosis of a stress fracture because of the rapidity of the bone changes. One week in a young child is usually sufficient to show an altered pattern consistent with the stress fracture rather than a tumour.

Infantile cortical hyperostosis or the 'battered baby' syndrome may be considered but with symptoms affecting only one bone in only one part of one limb both those diagnoses can be excluded without the necessity of radiographing the other parts of the child. If infantile cortical hyperostosis is suspected there is little urgency for further radiography, which when repeated after two or three weeks will confirm the diagnosis of a stress fracture (Figs. III.27 to III.29).

That there should be a different pattern of stress fractures in children as opposed to mature adults can be accepted in the same way that there is a difference between the greenstick and the ordinary fracture that occurs with injury. The stress fracture of childhood occurs during that time in which a greenstick fracture is found. Presumably it is this difference in bone strength and texture that alters the reaction to the stress that causes the fracture. Apart from the occasional finding of disuse of the limb preced-ing the stress fracture, it is rare to find any other history that might have a bearing on the condition. It is certainly impossible to inculpate osteoporosis or other debilitating

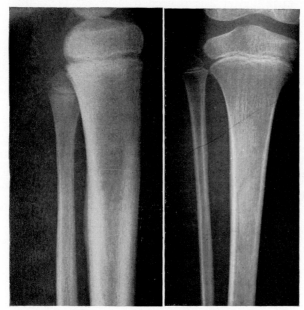

FIG. III.21   FIG. III.22

FIG. III.21   FIG. III.22

Figure III.21 shows a longitudinal stress fracture of the upper tibia in the radiograph of a boy aged 9 who only had a three days history of considerable pain in the upper shin. He had no injury. He was very tender in the upper shaft but an anteroposterior view taken later (FIG. III.22) suggests that the fracture, which can be seen in the posterior cortex in the lateral view, has extended downwards longitudinally. This patient made an uninterrupted recovery in a plaster.

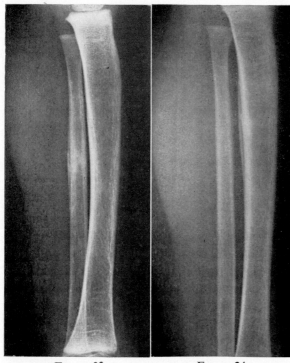

FIG. III.23   FIG. III.24

FIG. III.23   FIG. III.24

These are the radiographs of a boy aged about 2 who developed a stress fracture of the right fibula which healed satisfactorily (Fig. III.23). About eight months later he came back with more pain in the same leg. This pain was very similar to that which he had had previously, and at first the radiograph was normal but after a further month, during which he continued to limp, he was found to have a stress fracture (Fig III.24) in the upper third of the right tibia from which he made an excellent recovery.

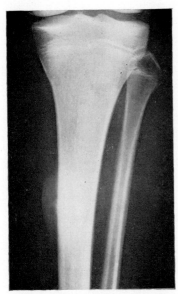

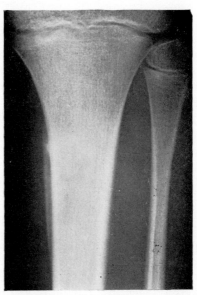

FIG. III.25

The radiograph of a child with an osteogenic sarcoma of the junction of the middle and upper thirds of the right tibia, later proven at biopsy. (Mr Rodney Sweetnam's case.)

FIG. III.26

The radiograph of a boy of 10 who was referred with a diagnosis of sarcoma. The stress fracture that he has is not dissimilar in this particular picture from the sarcoma shown in Figure III.25.

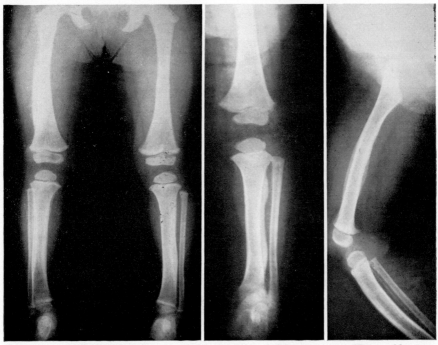

FIG. III.27   FIG. III.28   FIG. III.29

A girl of 3 years developed infantile cortical hyperostosis for no obvious reason. The radiological thickening of the bones might at first sight suggest healed, or healing, stress fractures but the multiplicity of lesions and the lack of internal callus allows easy distinction.

conditions as the cause of stress fractures in children as it might, perhaps, in the older adult.

An undiagnosed swelling in a child is always a cause for anxiety, especially if the radiograph does not exclude a tumour. Thus it is of great importance to arrange a biopsy if doubt exists. This is for two reasons: not only will it give a proper diagnosis, if indeed the child comes to operation without the true nature of the stress fracture becoming apparent, but, conversely, no tumour should ever be treated without a biopsy lest a stress fracture is, in fact, the real diagnosis. It is likely that some amputations have been done for simple stress fractures from which no biopsy has been taken to verify the diagnosis; it is not inconceivable that a cursory examination of the specimen might confirm the diagnosis, for the microscopical appearance of rapidly progressing callus in the young child can suggest the appearance of a sarcoma.

Oblique Stress Fractures of the Tibia

Oblique stress fractures of the tibia are most often found in young adults at about the age of 20. They occur particularly in athletes, either professional or part-time, and in military service recruits. Usually in the lowest third of the tibia, oblique stress fracture is sometimes seen in the uppermost third and rarely in the central shaft. The youngest patient who has been seen with an oblique stress fracture of the tibia was 14 years old; this was younger than the oldest compression stress fracture of the tibia seen in children. Both occur around that age according to skeletal maturity. Once the upper tibial epiphyses are closed or beginning to close, the oblique stress fracture starts to occur in place of the compression stress fracture seen in the child.

It is interesting that the compression stress fracture in the schoolboy athlete will have exactly the same symptomatology as the oblique fracture but the former is always in the uppermost third of the tibia; the oblique stress fracture is most common in the lowest third of the tibia.

The oldest patient seen with an oblique stress fracture was a man of 41 who was a marathon runner.

Because the young person is at risk for this fracture it is important to understand fully the type of activities that may produce it, not only from the point of view of sport but also from the way of life. The young man whose radiographs are shown in Figures III.30 and III.31 emphasised that, although his occupation was that of a bank clerk, he did in fact run at weekends and on such evenings as he could manage. Because the earliest symptoms are often said to be an ache in the evening, this aspect of recreation is very important or it might not be taken into account.

The progress of an oblique stress fracture of the tibia is well shown in Figures III.32 to III.37. The patient was a clerk, aged 21 and an athlete in his spare time. He had had shin soreness—which at one stage had been diagnosed as phlebitis—for two months and, when first seen, only a very slight haze of new bone could be seen on the medial aspect of the tibia in an anteroposterior view (Fig. III.32). However, after a further month the callus formation on the medial side was much more easily visible and there was perhaps the earliest sign of slight disruption of the medial cortex beneath this callus (Fig. III.33). Figure III.34 shows the fracture more clearly, and the fracture line can be seen running upwards and inwards from the medial cortex; it is seen better in the lateral view (Fig. III.35). At this time it was nearly four months since the onset

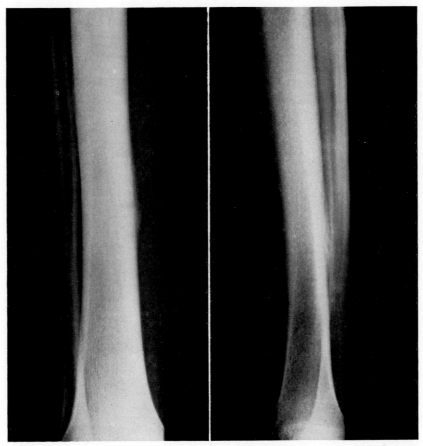

FIG. III.30   FIG. III.31

A man of 22 who ran in his spare time and at weekends attended an athlete's clinic with a painful lump at the junction of the middle and lowest third of his right shin which he had had for four weeks. Clinically the lump was felt on the posteromedial aspect of the subcutaneous border of the tibia. Figure III.30 shows the periosteal callus in a radiograph, and often this is all that is seen. However, in this patient the lateral radiograph (Fig. III.31) does show a crack in the posterior cortex running obliquely upwards.

E

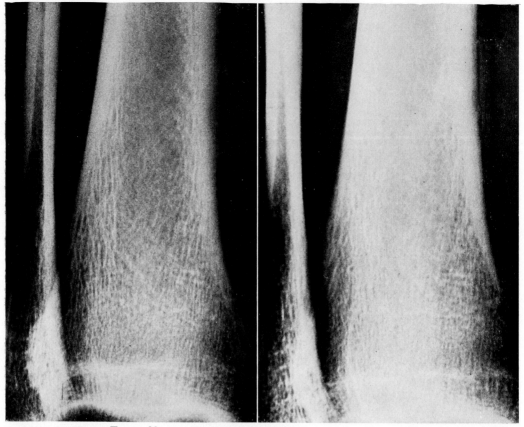

FIG. III.32   FIG. III.33

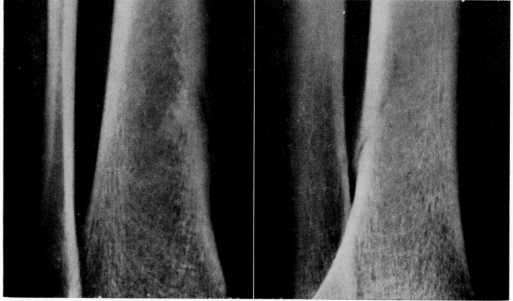

FIG. III.34   FIG. III.35

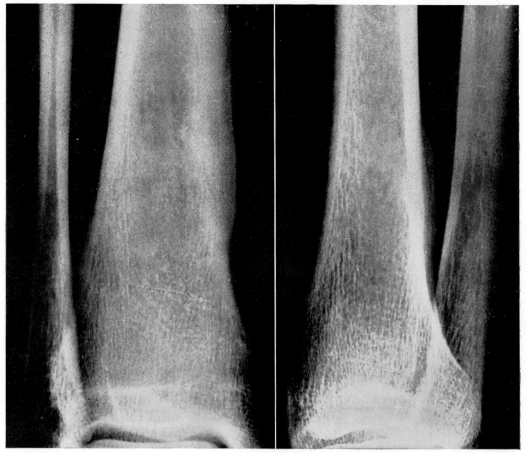

FIG. III.36   FIG. III.37

FIG. III.32 to FIG. III.37

A 21-year-old athlete attended two months after the onset of shin soreness. His radiograph in Figure III.32 shows a very faint haze of periosteal new bone on the medial side of the tibia. One month later the new bone formation is more obvious in Figure III.33 but there is no fracture line to be seen. A further three weeks later the fracture line can be seen but not very clearly in the antero-posterior radiograph in Figure III.34, but in the lateral projection taken at the same time the fracture is very much more obvious (Fig. III.35). It is now nearly four months since the onset of symptoms. Figures III.36 and III.37 show the final healing of this type of stress fracture in which only the postero-medial cortex of the tibia was involved. It is invariable that this fracture does not involve the whole of the shaft.

of symptoms. Figures III.36 and III.37 show final healing, at which stage the patient had returned to full training. The oblique stress fracture is very slow both to develop and to heal, and this must always be remembered when treating an athlete with this lesion.

Most oblique stress fractures occur in men with only about one out of 20 being seen in women. Probably this is because there are more male than female athletes; it is also important to realise that about one in five of patients with an oblique stress fracture of the tibia either has it bilaterally—simultaneously or at a later date—or has had a stress fracture elsewhere or even previously in the same tibia.

Figures III.38 to III.41 show very nicely the bilateral stress fracture of the lower third of the tibia. As is usual, one side develops more than the other and cuts down activity before the less well-developed fracture has time to progress to the same degree as the worst side. This patient also shows how difficult it is to see anything initially in the radiographs, which may be very slow to confirm the diagnosis.

About one in five patients with shin soreness have the stress fracture in the upper-most third of the tibia; at this site the fracture line goes obliquely downwards and laterally from the medial or posteromedial border of the tibia (Fig. III.42).

The younger patient often has more callus than has the mature adult, as is shown in Figure III.43. The swelling will also be increased locally, and the progress of the fracture to its full development and healing is quicker.

SYMPTOMS AND SIGNS

The history is usually long; very rarely is it only two or three weeks. It follows a similar, albeit slower, pattern to that of a stress fracture in the fibula but is less likely to stop activity altogether in the early stages since the ache does not become severe—indeed, it is often described as a soreness, hence the name of shin soreness. Care must be taken to find out if there have been similar symptoms either in the same leg or in the opposite leg concurrently or at a previous date. Figures III.44 and III.45 show the radiographs of the tibia of a girl of 20 (one of the few girls seen with this condition). The shin soreness of which she complained was high up the shin, medially and just below the knee; it was caused by an oblique stress fracture running downwards and laterally from the medial aspect of the uppermost third of the tibia. However, her history suggested that she had also had shin soreness the previous year and this assumption was supported by the buttressing of the tibial shaft, again posteromedially but in its lowest third.

The activity and occupation of the patient is important because many athletes are amateurs and play games at weekends or intermittently. They will give the typical history of pain—or soreness—after activity, coming on earlier and earlier during activity as time progresses. However, because of the intermittent nature of the sport of some athletes, the rest from sport during the week may prevent the symptoms developing very far and therefore they may complain of a moderately constant form of shin sore-ness which only gets worse very slowly. This will allow them to take part in sport on the Saturday, only to have it curtailed on the Sunday, to be fit, apparently, the following weekend, and for the same cycle of symptoms to recur each week; with each succeeding cycle the condition worsens.

The more professional athlete, who takes part in sport continuously, shows a slightly faster history with six weeks to two months being a reasonable average for the shin

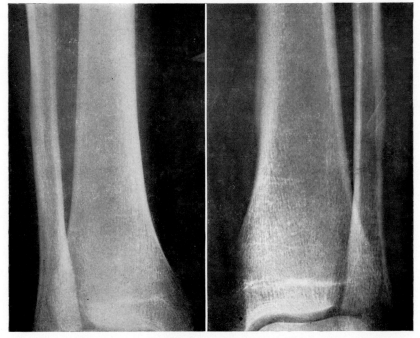

FIG. III.38   FIG. III.39

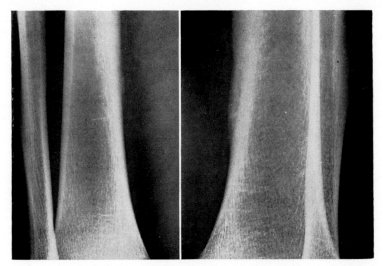

FIG. III.40   FIG. III.41

A medical student aged 25 developed pain in the right tibia. He was a keen cross-country runner. He was advised to rest, failed to do so and the pain recurred. He previously had had pain in the left tibia for seven months. Both his tibiae had stress fractures and failure to take proper advice of complete rest from sport had produced the second stress fracture by allowing that leg to do extra work in running. Figures III.39 and III.41 show the left leg with one month between radiographs, and Figures III.38 and III.40 show the right leg with a much smaller but equally definite stress fracture, again with one month between the radiographs. Note the marker in Figure III.38, which has accurately localised the site of the fracture after careful clinical appraisal.

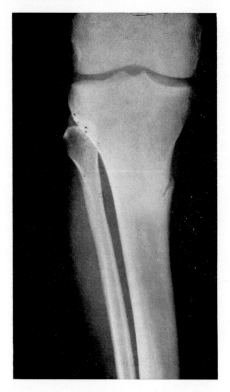

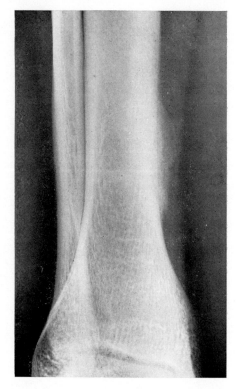

FIG. III.42

FIG. III.43

The classical stress fracture of the upper-most third of the tibia which occurred in a man of 18 who was a champion miler. He had a nine weeks history of 'torn muscle fibres', the pain of which had become gradually worse with increasing stiffness of the calf. When he attended for proper medical advice the radiograph was taken. The fracture runs downwards and laterally in this part of the tibia.

An athletic boy of 15 had a five weeks history of pain in the lower right tibia which had started after a cross-country run. It recurred the following day while training and had been painful ever since. The boy had noticed some swelling on the medial side of the tibia two days after the pain began. There was no history of injury. Examination showed that there was a bony hard and tender mass on the medial side of the lower third of the right tibia and the original radiograph shows a mass of periosteal new bone; no actual fracture line could be discerned in the cortex of the tibia. This amount of callus is unusual for the shin soreness type of oblique stress fracture except in the younger patient.

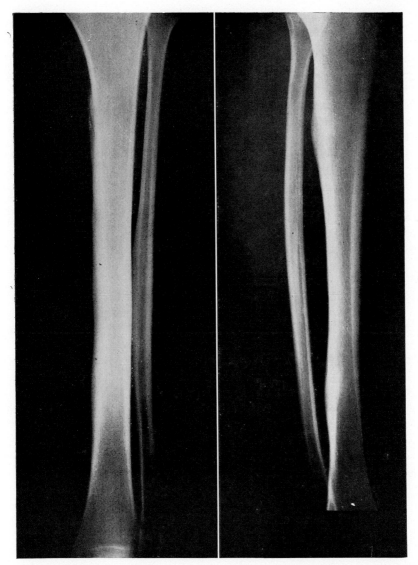

FIG. III.44   FIG. III.45

A girl aged 20 had the typical signs and symptoms of 'shin soreness' except that the site was in the uppermost third of the tibia. The fracture line runs downwards and inwards but is only through one cortex. There is evidence in the history and the radiographs that there had previously been a stress fracture in the lowest third of the same tibia.

soreness to develop to such an extent that athletics have to be abandoned and attention sought.

Always does the pain occur at first after sport as a dull ache or soreness in the shin. This is usually low down, and is often referred to the ankle or to the instep. When the pain is high, if the site of the fracture is at the top of the tibia, the pain can be referred down the shin.

There will be localised tenderness on examination; in the patient seeking advice early there may be some signs suggestive of mild inflammation such as heat, occasionally there can be felt a small bump or swelling on the medial tibia. If a swelling is felt it is hard, not soft. It is the same in the fibula. Being fusiform it blends into the shaft above and below, is difficult to feel and may easily be missed by the examining hand. It is never visible on inspection. If the patient is made to stand on tiptoe, or hop on tiptoe on the affected leg, very often the pain can be localised quite accurately (Figs. III.38 to III.41). Straining the tibia has never been found to be a useful manoeuvre.

Very rarely indeed an oblique stress fracture occurs in the centre of the tibia shaft (Figs. III.46 to III.49). This is a most important site because it is here that the very disabling transverse stress fracture will occur, as is described later in this chapter. Any symptom of a stress fracture at the centre of the tibial shaft warrants the immediate stopping of all sport and, preferably, a supporting plaster cast despite no radiological confirmation, which will be found after a further period of time. The young man illustrated in Figures III.46 to III.49 emphasises not only the importance of very careful examination and the difficulty in confirming the fractures radiologically but also that they may be bilateral, which is quite common, and especially at this site. In the radiographs, which are shown enlarged so that the slight thickening of the cortex of each tibia can be seen better, the first changes are not at all obvious and the radiographs could easily have been considered normal; that this was not so was due to the careful clinical appraisal before the radiographs were ordered. Any slipshod practice of having a radiograph taken 'to see if there is anything wrong' is even more liable to lead to disaster with a stress fracture than with most other lesions; radiography is there to confirm, not to make, the diagnosis.

RADIOLOGY

The oblique stress fracture of the tibia, as in many other stress fractures, is very slow to have radiological confirmation. Therefore the diagnosis must be clinical. Figure III.50 tells of the length of time taken for a stress fracture to be confirmed in a man of 25, who had had shin soreness for a year. The very considerable thickening of the tibial shaft in this patient is not all that uncommon and can be mistaken for that produced by an osteoid osteoma. The normal radiological anteroposterior or lateral projections may not help. Figure III.51 shows an oblique radiograph of the lowest third of the tibia in a boy of 17 in which the fracture line can be seen running upwards and inwards. Had this fracture line not been seen the picture would have been similar to that in Figure III.54, which is the radiograph of a girl who was in fact operated on for osteoid osteoma when she returned abroad, the correct diagnosis having been made previously. On the other hand, the fracture, when it is seen, may also remain very small, as is shown in Figure III.52. The appearance of these small lesions may suggest a diagnosis of 'periostitis' and often this is considered to be the cause of the condition; it has also been thought that the muscle attachment itself has been pulled up from the

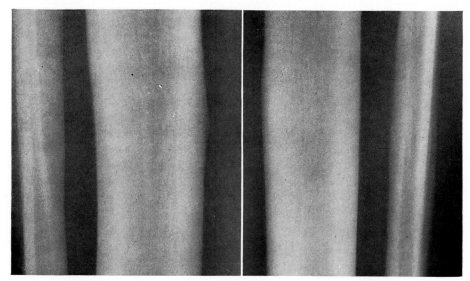

FIG. III.46   FIG. III.47

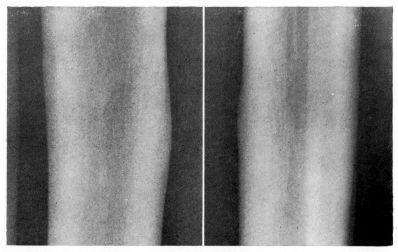

FIG. III.48   FIG. III.49

The transverse stress fracture of the centre shaft of the tibia is not the only stress fracture that will occur in that situation, and these radiographs show an oblique stress fracture at the centre of the tibial shafts. This athlete who kept in training by track running and sprinting developed pain in both tibiae at the same time one month before being seen. The original radiographs in Figures III.46 and III.47 show the right and left tibiae. The right tibia quite definitely shows a small bump of bone on the periosteal surface in the oblique view, and the left one also shows a similar but much less marked effect. One month later radiographs showed slight further development of the tibial swelling on the left (Fig. III.49) and the right (Fig. III.48) not only shows the progress of the swelling but the small thin fracture line can also be discerned. The fractures that occur in the midshaft of the tibia are difficult to diagnose radiologically when they are oblique. It is this condition that has caused difficulty in the understanding of stress fractures because very often all that has been seen is a thickening of the bone or a periosteal reaction with subperiosteal new bone formation.

periosteum to give rise to this appearance of periosteal new bone. Careful orientation in the taking of the radiographs of most patients will, almost invariably, show the fracture line, and thus it is unlikely that simple periostitis of a mechanical nature is the cause of shin soreness under any circumstances.

Perhaps the most typical finding in an ordinary radiograph of a man with pain in the lower shin is shown in Figure III.53, in which there is a small amount of new bone formation on the medial cortex of the lower third of the tibia. When the patient was first seen some four weeks after the onset of the symptoms this lump was no longer tender. He was 18 years old and had stopped his sport because the pain had prevented him running for a bus a few days after its onset. In the radiograph the healing stress fracture shows no fracture line; but careful inspection shows that the original line of the outside of the cortex is no longer clear-cut under the little lump of callus. This is a very important point in radiology. In all radiographs taken for this condition great care must be given to the viewing because of the minutiae of the findings. A naked electric light bulb must always be available as well as a viewing screen. The use of a magnifying glass is helpful.

Macrographs help sometimes; but properly positioned radiographs and a careful technique in exposure and development are just as good in the ordinary case.

DIAGNOSIS

The diagnosis of a stress fracture must be on clinical grounds, and any patient, including the athlete, must be considered to have a stress fracture without its being confirmed radiologically. Only in this way will the proper treatment be given at an early stage when it is most valuable. Clinically localised swelling may be found, but even in the absence of this and with only a vague tenderness over part of the shin the diagnosis should be made, provided the history of pain, aching or soreness at first after and then during activity, is present.

Again, it is important to emphasise that if the tenderness is in the centre shaft of the tibia there must be absolute rest from sport and a plaster cast must be applied until the diagnosis is established. The extremely rare oblique stress fracture that does occur in the central third of the tibia (Figs. III.46 to III.49) should be treated in the same way although it is perhaps less sinister in its complications.

The great thickening of the cortex that is quite often found, especially in the less severe but more chronic tibial stress fracture, has led to the diagnoses of other conditions, such as osteoid osteoma (Fig. III.54). Figure III.55 shows the initial radiograph of a naval cadet which could be mistaken for 'periostitis', particularly if the fracture line did not show—as it does here—in the oblique view. In the standard views the fracture line, running upwards and inwards, did not show and the irregularity of the new bone formation will not suggest a stress fracture unless the condition is well understood.

When the stress fracture occurs in the uppermost third of the tibia (Figs. III.56 and III.57) it can occasionally make the unwary clinician consider that there is an internal derangement of the knee, particularly as symptoms occur just below the medial joint line, with the result that an undamaged medial meniscus is removed.

Figures III.55 and III.56 also bear out the fact that the young man recently enlisted into military service gets the same stress fracture as does the athlete; it is the emphasis on physical exercise in the early stages of training that leads to the fracture.

FIG. III.50

The shin soreness stress fracture may take a long time to develop and a long time to show radiologically. This man of 25, an athlete who specialised in running, had had gradual onset of pain in the lower third of his tibia over one year which was always eased by rest. When seen at the end of that time he was tender at the site of the pain. The radiograph shows the thickened cortex and the fracture line. Compare this with the very similar appearance in Figure III.51.

FIG. III.51

A stress fracture in a boy of 17 who had shin soreness. In the radiograph the fracture line can just be seen going up through a healed thickened cortex. It is fortunate that the beam of the x-ray has gone through the original fracture line otherwise it would not have been seen. This picture should be compared to that in Figure III.54. This appearance is typical of a healed shin soreness type of stress fracture.

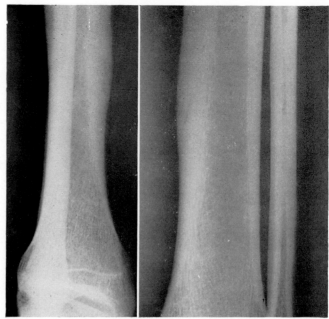

FIG. III.50   FIG. III.51

FIG. III.52

When it appears, the radiological lesion may be minute. This athlete, a man of 27, had had pain in the left shin in a six-mile race which had come on gradually. He was found to have a painful and tender lump almost at the junction of the middle and lowest third of the tibia which could just be seen in the radiograph. He remained painful at this site for two months before it was healed.

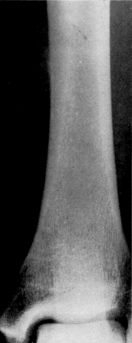

FIG. III.52

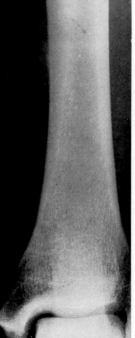

FIG. III.53

An engineering student aged 18, who was a cross-country runner and a miler. He was in full training and very fit when he developed shin soreness early in the new year. The pain was insidious in origin. It had started after he had been running; a few days later he tried to run for a bus and found he could not do so. Examination four weeks after the onset of symptoms showed a lump at the site of the lesion which was no longer tender. The radiograph at the same time showed a small area of new bone formation which is far less and far more discrete than that shown in Figure III.43.

FIG. III.54

A girl was diagnosed as having had a stress fracture of the tibia. The thickening of the cortex was all that could be seen in the radiographs. She left England and went back to her own country where an operation was done on the assumption that she had an osteoid osteoma because she was still getting slight symptoms. No osteoid osteoma was discovered but the wound went septic and this interference on a misdiagnosis was disastrous to the patient.

FIG. III.55

A naval cadet who was the cross-country champion developed pain in the lowest third of the right tibia after he had run 12 miles. The following day he said he was normal in regard to walking but got pain standing on tiptoe. Enquiry showed that he had developed similar symptoms previously which had come and gone over four months. Examination showed slight tenderness over the lower third of the right subcutaneous surface of the tibia and on its medial border. There was a firm, painless swelling at that area. The radiograph shows the stress fracture but only in the oblique view, all others showing thickening of the cortex or a little subperiosteal new bone only. One year previously he had had a similar fracture of the left tibia.

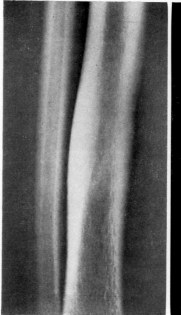 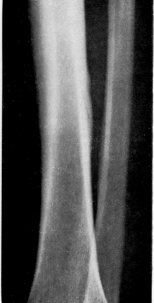

FIG. III.54   FIG. III.55

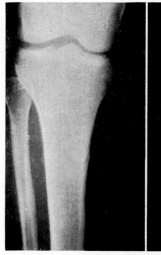 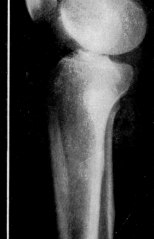

FIG. III.56   FIG. III.57

Whether the oblique stress fracture is in the upper or lower part of the tibia the symptoms can be present for a long time before radiographic changes occur. A marine aged 17 who had been in the service for ten months, had had nine weeks pain on the medial border of the upper right tibia of which he had complained after the first three days. Although tenderness had been found no change had been seen in the radiograph then or a month later and it was only when the radiograph in Figure III.56 was taken nine weeks after the onset of symptoms that the fracture could be seen in the uppermost third of the tibia running downwards and laterally through the medial cortex. The lateral view could still be considered normal although there was a suggestion of a faint periosteal thickening with bone formation in one area corresponding to the level of the fracture (Fig. III.57).

In the diagnosis of the oblique stress fracture of the tibia the radiographs never show involvement of both cortices. A different form of stress fracture occurs in the middle-aged and older age groups; this is a compression stress fracture, which can usually be differentiated by the age and activity of the patient. Such compression stress fractures are described later in this chapter and in Chapter Four.

Stress fractures of the fibula can mislead despite the fact that they are on the lateral side of the ankle, or shin, if the fracture is high in the fibula. This may cause difficulty, but only in the early stages because it is then that the symptoms can be vague and poorly localised and are often said to be in the 'front of the ankle'. Furthermore, the athlete has often been conditioned by a trainer to believe his symptoms are coming from a specific place, which does not help, and which necessitates a very careful painstaking examination.

TREATMENT

The treatment of the oblique stress fracture of the tibia is rest, continuous and uninterrupted, for at least one month. At the end of that time the progress of the fracture healing is assessed. The professional athlete may be allowed to exercise the other parts of the affected leg, if this is clinically aceptable and if it causes no pain at the fracture site. Once union is occurring the exercise is graded so that it is insufficient to cause any symptoms in the healing fracture. If the fracture is not yet healed enough, or if the activity is too great, some aching will occur and exercise must be stopped before harm is done. If any ache occurs at any time further rest must be instituted immediately. In other words, the bone must be allowed to heal sufficiently so that gentle exercise will not cause further disruption or stressing of the fracture site.

Elastic adhesive strapping is usually all that is necessary for supporting the shin. This must be carefully applied from the toes upwards with a uniform tension of the strapping as it is applied. With this, the weekend athlete may normally continue to do his work and to commute to and from the office but he must understand the necessity of not causing pain at the site of the fracture.

The condition occasionally necessitates a below-knee walking plaster, particularly to keep the industrious athlete at rest; with this, or with adhesive strapping, the other limbs must be exercised to the full so that there is no weakening in general nor loss of tone. The affected leg must also be exercised, but not while weight-bearing because this is too strenuous and causes pain by stressing the fracture site. Thigh, knee and foot exercises will help to maintain tone. Walking in the supporting plaster is allowed, provided that it is not done to excess so that it causes pain.

Unfortunately most advice, given on the track or in the training quarters, for so-called pulled muscles or inflammations will be deleterious to the athlete with a stress fracture. Figures III.58 to III.60 show a sequence of radiographs that might at first seem to confirm a 'mild inflammation' with which diagnosis, the patient, badly treated and insufficiently rested, gets recurrence after recurrence of the shin soreness and loses a whole season of sport.

DISCUSSION

The importance of the oblique stress fracture is that it affects young people in the prime of life and that, by misdiagnosis and ill-treatment, a promising career may be spoilt at the worst or a season's pleasurable activity ruined at the least.

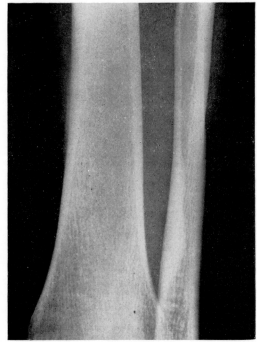

FIG. III.58

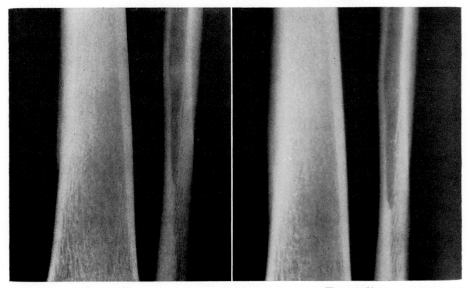

FIG. III.59   FIG. III.60

A schoolboy of 17 who did much running, had pain in the left tibia for 10 days and was referred to hospital. The radiograph shown in Figure III.58 was taken when he was seen and shows a very faint periosteal reaction. The radiograph after a further month (Fig. III.59) shows more reaction and the suggestion of a crack in the cortex. The final radiograph, some months later (Fig. III.60), shows the healed area in which the fracture line can still just be seen under the callus.

Because the symptoms are mild initially, respond rapidly to rest, but recur again if the rest is not long enough, the cycle of pain, rest, activity and then more pain may continue for many weeks or months before the patient seeks proper medical advice and obtains correct treatment. By this time it is often too late for the athlete to return to full fitness for the particular season of sport concerned.

Aches or pains in the shin of an athlete are often felt lower down the leg. If they occur in the upper shin, the pain may be considered to be referred from the knee. The active young man must have a very careful clinical examination after the history has been gone into in great detail. Ready-made explanations of a twist, a jar, a jolt should not be accepted without further enquiry to make quite certain that such an injury did, in fact, occur. The athlete in particular will often think that an injury must have occurred to account for the pain.

After the history has been taken the examination must be painstaking and slow. The patient's preconceived diagnosis may divert attention from the real cause. This is what happened when 'shin soreness' originated as a diagnosis in sport and it was thought to be a condition amenable to active treatment, embrocations, exercises, massage and so on. There could hardly be worse treatment for this stress fracture.

Once the diagnosis has been made correctly it is essential to give a careful explanation to the athlete so that he understands fully what is going on, otherwise the advice on treatment, although apparently accepted, may be altered by the athlete visiting some source of fringe medicine and being told that he must 'run it off'. When the clinical assessment of the patient's general attitude is such that it is felt that elastic adhesive strapping and the advice to rest are not strong enough measures, then without any doubt a below-knee walking plaster should be used (and this is quite sufficient also for the shin soreness stress fracture in the uppermost third of the tibia) and rest is thus ensured. In the early stress fracture at least three to four weeks of complete rest must be given according to the length and severity of the symptoms when the patient first attended. At the end of this time rest must be continued if there are still symptoms from the stress fracture or if tenderness is still present. Sometimes, to be really safe, it is necessary to await the radiological evidence of healing.

This, however, is not all. The return to full activity or training must be gradual. The athlete must be told to start gentle running or skipping, and no competitive activity is allowed until full painless function has returned. Excessive endeavours to catch up will often bring back the symptoms if the stress fracture has not healed strongly.

If a plaster cast has been used the time to get back to full training must be taken even more cautiously because the immobilisation in plaster will have done nothing to strengthen the tibia as a whole. Indeed it will only maintain its strength if the rest of the leg is properly exercised.

The aetiology of this particular stress fracture is most interesting as it occurs in young men and women who, being athletic or in military service, represent the most healthy of their age group. It is this particular aspect of the oblique stress fracture which lends the greatest support to the assumption that the fracture is not in any way pathological nor caused through disease or inherent weakness of bone, either local or general. Further, in stress fractures of the fibula it has been shown that the movement of the fibula that occurs with ordinary muscular activity is quite considerable. Although the tibia is a very much stronger bone than the fibula the same forces must also apply to the tibia; it is therefore to be expected that the oblique crack should appear on the medial side of the bone which is the side that is distracted by the muscle pull. It is a bending movement of the bone that produces the fracture and it is not the jarring of each footfall.

Prevention of this fracture should include the proper understanding of the cause and include certain practices of which proper graduated training must take first place. It is also important to recognise that, when a young service recruit starts heavy training, such as long runs, the footwear at first should have thick soles of soft material. Such shoes should also be worn for athletes who wish to train on hard roads in place of a soft track. The thick sole allows the contraction of the muscles resisting each footfall to be buffered and more gradual than if the sole is thin and hard.

With training, muscle power increases rapidly but the increase in bone strength takes a great deal longer and time must be allowed for this to happen or, inevitably, the stresses on the bone will become greater than those it has strength to resist and a stress fracture will occur.

Compression Stress Fractures in Adults

It is extremely rare to find this condition under the age of 50 and, although it does occur in men, it is again very rare without some obvious predisposing cause. About half the women who have compression stress fractures of the tibia also have a stress fracture of the fibula at the same level. About one in five of the stress fractures of the tibia are of this compression variety and, of these, about one in ten is in a man, but men are rarely seen with the simultaneous stress fracture of the tibia and fibula which is dealt with in Chapter Four. The average age of the patients with compression stress fractures of the tibia is in the late sixties; it has been seen up to the age of 90 and doubtless could be found at an even older age but the fragility of the bone from osteoporosis is such that it begins to make the diagnosis difficult. Usually the fracture is in the lowest third of the tibia but it does occur in the uppermost third and, in the very elderly, in the centre shaft.

Symptoms and Signs

The classical presentation of this condition is of 'chronic' pain in the ankle with radiological confirmation of the fracture that is very slow to develop (Figs. III.61 to III.64). The patient will complain that she has had pain in the ankle for many weeks. This may be associated with swelling of which the patient may also complain; both the pain and swelling are worse with activity. Sometimes the pain at night is severe. Treatment has usually been given for various diagnoses quite commonly including 'phlebitis' but understandably to no avail. The past history may show some unusual activity to have been present as was the case in Figures III.65 to III.75. Sometimes the patient will have had some condition, such as bed rest, that has allowed the bone to lose some of its strength, as is shown in Figures III.61 and III.69. In some of the older patients the history may indicate that there has been either a cause for osteoporosis or that there have been symptoms in the past attributable to the secondary effects of this condition. Some of the patients will complain of very severe pain indeed and their attendance may be as an emergency, particularly where the fracture has been in the centre of the tibial shaft and caused some displacement. This type is rare in the younger patients but more common the older they get (Fig. III.70).

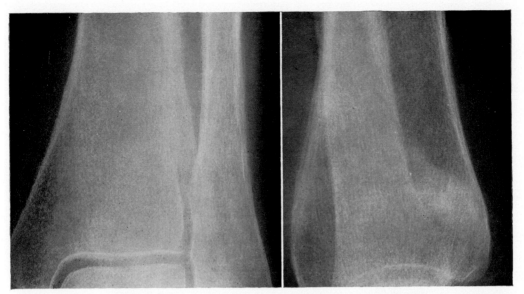

FIG. III.61   FIG. III.62

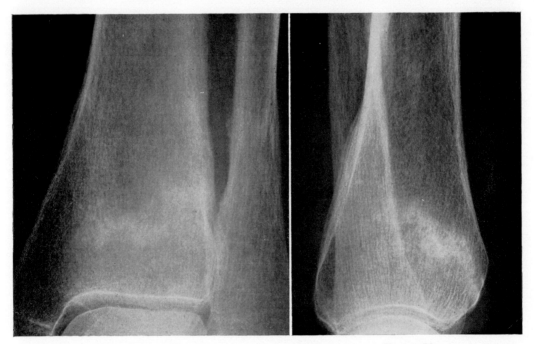

FIG. III.63   FIG. III.64

A 69-year-old lady had had a Smith-Petersen pinning operation for a fracture of the left femoral neck. Three months later, having been by then walking for two months, she developed pain above the ankle with no changes in the radiographs of the tibia. It was not for two months that the radiographs (Figs. III.61 and III.62) showed the faint haze of internal callus. After a further month this was much more evident (Figs. III.63 and III.64). This patient shows that it may take a very long time for the radiological changes to confirm a compression stress fracture. Her symptoms continued for a further three months.

F

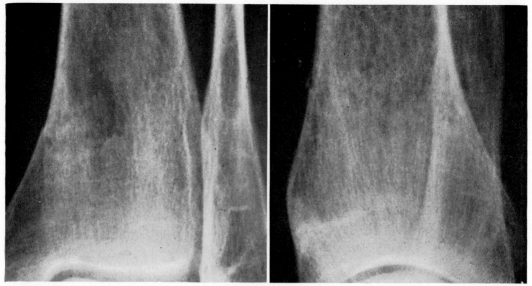

FIG. III.65

FIG. III.66

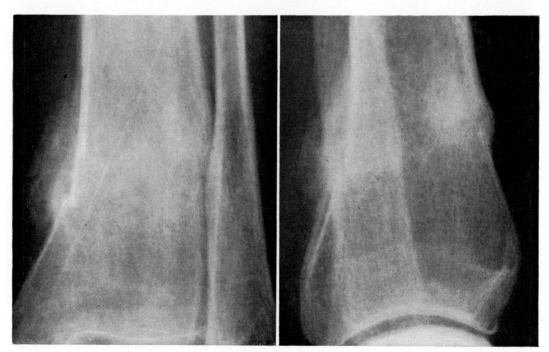

FIG. III.67

FIG. III.68

A woman who believed she was a stork stood on one leg for long periods in what was then called a lunatic asylum. One day she was found to be unable to walk and was thought to have sustained a bee sting because the leg was red and swollen. However, the radiographs showed a typical compression stress fracture of the lowest third of the tibia on which she was wont to stand (Figs. III.65 and III.66). There was little displacement but there was a haze of internal callus across the tibia at the level of the fracture. Later, considerable callus developed outside the cortex as well as inside it (Figs. III.67 and III.68). She made a complete recovery.

If the fracture is in the lowest third of the tibia—and two out of three are at this site—the pain is less severe than from those which occur in the midshaft or in the uppermost third of the tibia where the strain upon the fracture is greater.

The fracture at the top of the tibia can be similar to that in the child, again emphasising the similarity between certain stress fractures in children and in late adult life. Figures III.71 and III.72 show such a stress fracture in the uppermost third of the tibia in a woman of 57 who had developed sudden pain in the knee but did not recall any injury. This patient also shows that although the pain was felt in the knee there was no effusion on examination. In six weeks time, and with no treatment, she was quite better.

RADIOLOGY

The problem of confirming the diagnosis of compression stress fracture is that very often the radiological changes are extremely late so that, by the time they are ultimately shown, many patients are already improving, if not free of symptoms. This means that if successive radiological examinations are not done the true diagnosis may never be made, or at best never confirmed radiologically. Figures III.73 and III.74 show the radiographs of one of the few men who developed this fracture above the ankle. In the first anteroposterior radiograph, some five weeks after his symptoms had started, little if anything can be discerned except perhaps a slight rarefaction just above the medial malleolus (Fig. III.73). He was treated by rest and support for the diagnosis of a thrombosed vein and he was given Butazolidin. One month later the compression stress fracture of the lower tibia was more easily visible with a haze of internal callus on its lateral aspect and the line of the fracture on the medial side being slightly more obvious.

DIAGNOSIS

The slow development of radiological changes makes it most important that the condition be fully understood so that when a patient does present with a stress fracture, and this applies particularly to the elderly, it must be recognised. The history of pain on activity—even if its onset was abrupt—with no injury and of worsening of the pain with further activity is, as usual, an indication of a stress in bone. Careful taking of the history to find out exactly how the pain affects the patient and its association with rest and exercise, followed by a very careful clinical examination, will enable the clinical diagnosis to be made. The association of swelling of the affected part must not be allowed to confuse. In the early stages of the fracture the swelling comes and goes with the pain and, therefore, with activity; later the swelling may be present the whole time.

There are many other conditions which simulate this stress fracture, from osteoarthritis of the neighbouring joint to vascular disease, including claudication and phlebitis. Any form of general arthritic condition may mask the onset of pain, which, when it occurs, is ascribed to 'rheumatism'. Carcinomatosis with secondaries in the tibia is seen occasionally. It can be differentiated by the history because the pain starts as an ache without the same relationship to activity. It must be remembered, however, that if there is a defect in the bone which weakens it sufficiently the symptoms may mimic those of a stress fracture absolutely because the bone is in fact gradually fracturing through a pathological lesion. At this stage radiography will always disclose

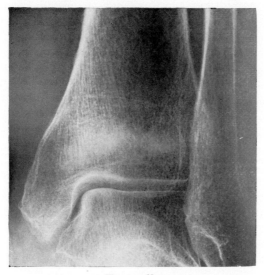

FIG. III.69   FIG. III.70

FIG. III.69   The typical radiological appearance of a compression stress fracture in the lower end of the tibia in a woman of 78. The cloud of internal callus can be seen passing across the expanded lower end of the tibia but the cortex on either side does not seem to have been involved.

FIG. III.70   This is the radiograph of a woman of 80 who complained of a tender swelling of the right shin which she had had for six weeks and which, for the last two weeks, had prevented her walking because it had become too painful. She was treated by plaster cast for three weeks followed by firm bandaging for a further seven weeks. The stress fracture in the middle third of the tibia has compressed slightly but has united with no angulation of note despite the fact that the patient continued to walk on it for some while without any protection.

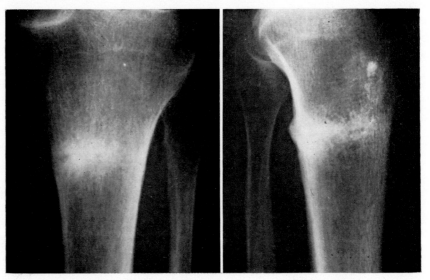

FIG. III.71   FIG. III.72

The radiographs of a woman of 57 who had a sudden pain in the right knee and difficulty in walking but had no injury. She attended for advice at hospital some six weeks later when the right knee showed a full range of movement and no effusion. She had slight tenderness and she walked with a limp. She has a compression stress fracture of the upper third of the right tibia which is remarkably like that seen in a child.

the lesion. Osteoporosis is present in most patients with this form of fracture and in all in the older age group. Varicose veins may give rise to ulcers, and the pain from the ulcer may mask the pain from a stress fracture of the bone beneath the ulcer. The pain and swelling that goes with gout may be difficult to distinguish from a stress fracture, but can be excluded by the routine serological tests. Sometimes the acute onset and the considerable swelling that this stress fracture can produce, combined with the finding of poor vascularity, may suggest bone infection, but without fever. Other vascular conditions can be excluded by careful examination and investigation.

One important aspect of this, or any other, stress fracture in the elderly is that all too often the patient has multiple, if mild, general aches, pains, 'muscular rheumatism' and so on; this means that a new symptom may be buried under a veritable avalanche of other complaints and, unless great patience is used, the typical history of the new pain in its own right may well be left undiscovered.

TREATMENT

In the very old patient with a fracture of the shaft of the tibia, such as is shown in Figures III.75 and III.76, it may be necessary to use internal fixation, not only to achieve fixation of the fragments but also in order to keep the patient mobile. Bed rest—which the symptoms often induce—is the worst treatment for this condition, although to the elderly patient staying in bed seems preferable to hobbling painfully around the home. Other patients, particularly those with the fractures near the knee, may need plaster immobilisation and if this is used it should not be in the form of a plaster cylinder from groin to ankle but should include the foot, otherwise, being a compression fracture, weight-bearing still causes pain. Usually, however, some simple supportive bandaging, such as elastic adhesive bandage or two layers of a firm circular compression bandage, is sufficient to allow the patient to continue to walk. The very elderly will need a walking aid, from a stick to a frame. The compression stress fractures of the tibia only are never as difficult to treat as those in which the tibia and fibula are both involved (Chapter Four), even though the pain is as severe.

DISCUSSION

Compression stress fractures are caused by excessive stress causing the bone to fail. At first, as in the distraction stress fracture, the fracture is at molecular level, later it involves trabeculae so that there is a physical inflammation with all its consequences including early attempts at repair. This accounts for the early haze of internal callus, which is the first radiological sign.

Generalised osteoporosis undoubtedly plays a part in the compression stress fracture of the tibia in the older patient (Figs. III.75 and 76). This is why activity is not only encouraged but insisted upon because decubitus gives rise to more osteoporosis. Although many of these stress fractures have occurred in patients between 50 and 60 they are most common in later life, with the average age for the whole group being about 70 years.

The treatment of the stress fracture of the shaft of the tibia in the elderly must be as radical as possible, and there should be no hesitation in using intramedullary fixation rather than a cumbersome plaster cast so that the patient can be returned to the activities of daily living with the least delay.

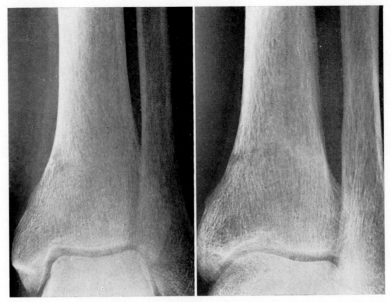

FIG. III.73   FIG. III.74

A man of 68 noticed a sudden onset of swelling of the ankle with some pain which his doctor thought might have been caused by a deep vein thrombosis. He was given Butazolidin 100 mg three times a day. This caused a reaction and was stopped, and the leg was strapped and five weeks later he had the first radiograph taken in which there is little to be seen except slight rarefaction around the medial border of the tibia above the medial malleolus (Fig. III.73). However, after a further four weeks the internal callus can be seen on the lateral side of the shaft of the tibia just above the ankle and the medial continuation of the fracture is more obvious (Fig. III.74).

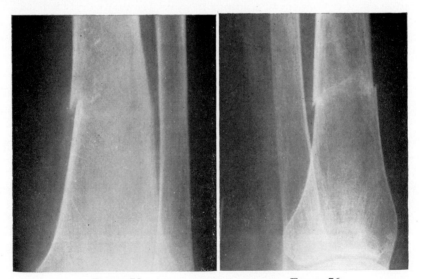

FIG. III.75   FIG. III.76

A woman of 85 had been bedridden for five years with an osteoarthritic hip which had become stiff in a very deformed position. An osteotomy produced a satisfactory result and she was allowed up, weight-bearing, three months after operation. Two months after this she developed a stress fracture in the lowest third of the tibia, as shown in the radiographs. Later she was also to develop a stress fracture in the pubis. Both stress fractures healed without incident.

Longitudinal Stress Fractures of the Tibia

A longitudinal stress fracture may involve half or more of the shaft of a long bone and is most often seen in the tibia; it does occur rarely in the femur, the metatarsal shaft, and the child's fibula. It can be most misleading in symptoms, signs and radiographic appearances and needs to be fully understood before it can be diagnosed early in its course.

This stress fracture forms about 10 per cent of stress fractures seen in the tibia. It is seen from childhood (see page 50) to senescence, and at both extremes it is more difficult to diagnose. The oldest patient seen with this fracture was 76, but the average age of occurrence in the adult is around 50. It is twice as common in women as in men; it can occur in the athlete.

The stress fracture appears, radiologically, almost to be an extension proximally (or distally sometimes) of the ordinary oblique stress fracture of shin soreness but it is always more difficult to diagnose and slower in its development.

SYMPTOMS AND SIGNS

The history, even in the younger adult, can be lengthy. It is insidious in origin. The ache, noticed some weeks or months before attendance, is in the shin. It comes on with activity, at first only present when the patient is tired, then during activity, and later present the whole time. The intensity gradually increases until it prevents sleep (Figs. III.77 to III.79). Sport or energetic activity is impossible (Figs. III.80 to III.82).

Occasionally, and particularly in the older patient, severe symptoms come on suddenly.

Sometimes a patient who has had a mild aching in the shin for several weeks will cause the symptoms to become severe by a trivial stumble. The ache can be less obvious to the patient than is the swelling which, when noticed in the lower calf and shin, may be the presenting complaint and mislead the clinician; especially is this so if there is any other local condition to which the swelling might be attributed, such as varicose veins (Figs. III.83 to III.86).

As in all stress fractures, the activity of the patient is very important; Figures III.87 and III.88 show the radiographs of a patient who had recently taken up a very active job entailing much walking.

The clinical examination will reveal a point of tenderness in the shin, about usually the junction of the middle and lowest third, particularly on the subcutaneous border, but there is also general tenderness in the calf and further up the shin. Careful deep examination, particularly through the muscles of the calf, will find this tenderness. At rest, movement of the foot, ankle and knee will be full and free with no limitation of movement unless arthritis or some other local condition prevents this, which can mislead the unwary observer. Pain, arising in the hip or knee, and which is not uncommon in the older group, may detract from the careful examination of the calf and consideration to be referred. Very often varicose veins are present and indicted for the ache simply because they are present. The younger patient, and particularly the athlete, will show less swelling than in the older person and the tenderness may be more localised than it is in the older patient, with a more swollen leg. Later a hard lump may be felt on the tibia but this is by no means as constant as that found in the oblique stress fracture. Heat, redness, swelling and tenderness around the fracture

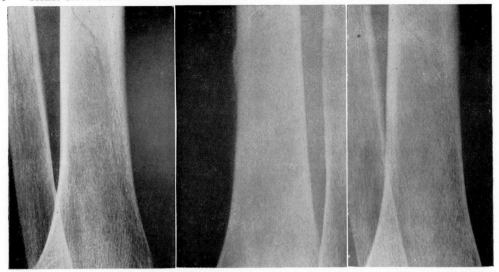

FIG. III.77   FIG. III.78   FIG. III.79

A woman of 76 felt a snap in her leg while she was walking quite normally up some steps. She was certain that she had not fallen nor even tripped on anything. The longitudinal stress fracture can be seen in the initial radiograph (Fig. III.77) which was taken on the same day, and in Figures III.78 and III.79 two months after the onset of symptoms when the radiographs show that the fracture line is still visible but only in the lateral view. There is a little callus only to be seen in the anteroposterior view. The lack of history, unusual for stress fractures in general, is more common with this stress fracture than any other.

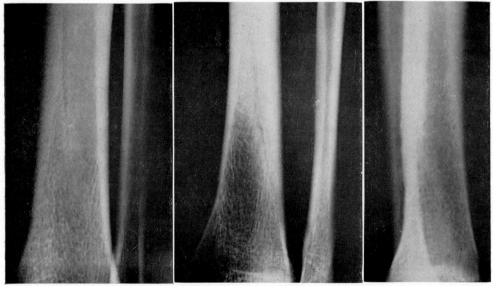

FIG. III.80   FIG. III.81   FIG. III.82

An athlete aged 19 had three months pain in his shin. Clinically it was so typical of shin soreness that radiographs were repeated until the fracture line was seen, but it was a longitudinal stress fracture that appeared. Elastic adhesive strapping and rest from sport had been his treatment. It is interesting that the fracture line when first seen in a macrograph was reported to be an artefact (Fig. III.80). Figures III.81 and III.82 show the tibia five weeks after the first radiograph when the fracture line is obvious. It runs longitudinally up the tibial shaft. The anterior cortex of the tibia in the lateral view shows no abnormality (Fig. III.82).

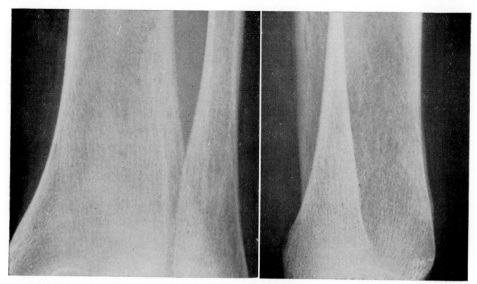

FIG. III.83   FIG. III.84

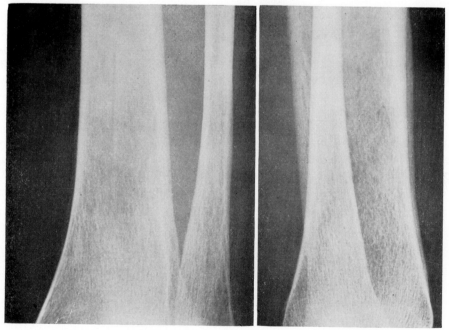

FIG. III.85   FIG. III.86

A woman of 61 had three months pain in the shin which was diagnosed by her clinician as a tibial periostitis of unknown origin. She was extensively investigated to no effect, and, in Figures III.83 and III.84 there is only to be seen a little periosteal new bone formation in the lateral projection of the radiographs. Two weeks later the periosteal reaction was more extensive (Figs. III.85 and III.86) and a longitudinal fracture line in the anterior cortex of the tibia is visible in the anteroposterior radiograph. There is no fracture in the posterior cortex and there is no callus to be seen there.

are at times present, particularly in those patients with a very long history, which can simulate osteomyelitis (Figs. III.89 and III.90). Forced distraction or bending of the tibia rarely produces the pain.

RADIOLOGY

The radiographs can be very slow to confirm a longitudinal stress fracture and the fracture line that is eventually seen running up the shaft of the tibia may take three months or more to show. Figures III.80 to III.82 are the radiographs of a young man who was diagnosed clinically as having an oblique stress fracture—or shin soreness— which he had developed while running. Despite careful and repeated radiography it was at 13 weeks after the onset of symptoms that the ordinary radiographs showed the longitudinal stress fracture. However, five weeks earlier the diagnosis had been made on clinical grounds and when the normal radiograph showed no fracture a macrograph was fortunately taken in such a position that the fracture showed (Fig. III.80). It is unusual that a macrograph is so helpful but this serves as an excellent demonstration of how long ordinary radiology may take to find confirmation of the fracture.

Often the radiological confirmation is absent and some other diagnosis is made, as happened to the patient whose radiographs are shown in Figures III.83 to III.86. Here the periosteal reaction on the creast of the tibia was taken to be a 'periostitis'. It is, of course, necessary for the beam of the X-ray tube to pass either tangentially across the fracture, where it runs up the cortex of the tibia so as to show this apparent periosteal new bone formation, or to pass accurately through the crack at right angles to the cortex in whichever direction the break may happen to lie (Figs. III.91 and III.92). Standard views should not be accepted if they fail to confirm the fracture; radiographs must be taken at oblique angles and also repeated after a period of time. In contra-distinction to the slowness of most longitudinal stress fractures to show in radiographs those with a sudden onset are usually visible in radiographs at an early stage, if not at once. Compare the radiographs in Figures III.93 and III.77 of which both patients had had a sudden onset of pain, but it is possible to consider that the stress fracture had been present previously and a sudden extension of the fracture occurred to cause pain. This is sometimes the cause of an abrupt onset of symptoms in stress fractures of the fibula and in some other bones.

DIAGNOSIS

The diagnosis is made on the history and clinical examination despite the negative radiological findings. Treatment must then be given with every confidence, which, if started sufficiently early in the course of the fracture, may achieve healing of the stress fracture without there ever being confirmation from the radiographs. This is because the early radiological signs may be very difficult to obtain, so that the fracture passes unnoticed.

The differential diagnosis can cause problems if a careful history and clinical examina-tion is not allowed to be influenced by other obvious pathology of the part. Both the patients in Figures III.80 to III.86 had had a hot red swelling over the lower shin and were diagnosed as suffering from a subacute osteomyelitis—despite a normal tempera-ture—and 'periostitis' respectively. Further radiographs after the pain and swelling had subsided with the bed rest revealed the true state of affairs.

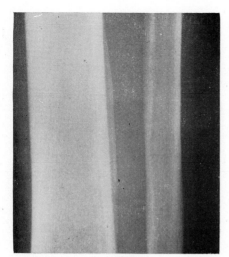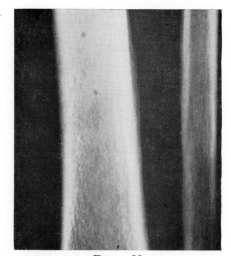

FIG. III.87   FIG. III.88

A woman of 48 noticed pain in the lower leg after much unaccustomed walking, having taken up a new occupation. Several weeks after the onset of this pain radiographs showed callus towards the back of the tibia (Fig. III.87). The radiograph in Figure III.88 was taken after a further two weeks. The fracture does not show clearly because it runs in the plane of the radiograph.

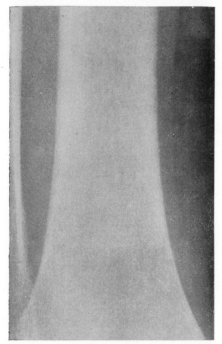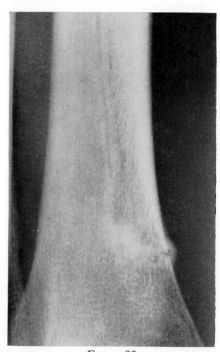

FIG. III.89   FIG. III.90

A middle-aged woman complained of pain, swelling and tenderness above the ankle and she was thought to have osteomyelitis. The initial radiograph (Fig. III.89) showed a hazy translucent area in the lower medial cortex of the tibia, which appeared to confirm the clinical diagnosis. After four weeks the fracture can be seen running as a double line up the tibia (Fig. III.90). It appears thus because the fracture runs through both the anterior and the posterior tibial cortex.

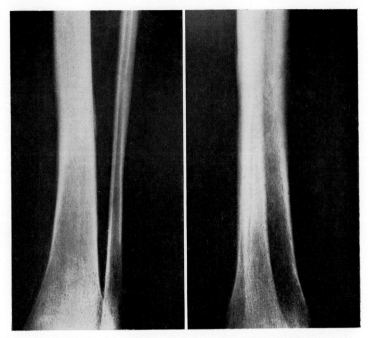

FIG. III.91   FIG. III.92

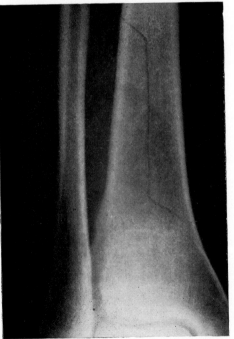

FIG. III.93

Figure III.91 shows the radiograph of a woman of 57 who had a six weeks history of pain in the lower left shin which spread to the ankle and which was worse on walking. She had had no injury but she had had some arthritis in the left knee. She was found to have swelling over the lower third of the left calf and shin with tenderness over both tibia and fibula. The radiograph showed a typical longitudinal stress fracture in which the periosteal reaction on the surface of the bone was first noted. In the lateral radiograph (Fig. III.92) the fracture line can be seen running up from the lower posterior cortex and then in the upper part running anteriorly and superiorly to the anterior cortex. This patient was treated in a below-knee walking plaster in which she made an excellent recovery. The fine fracture line is seen best in its upper part because here the x-ray beam passed perpendicularly through it.

FIG. III.93

A man of 64 was lifting a heavy table and turned around with his weight on the right leg. He heard a crack and a few minutes later (but not immediately) developed a pain in the leg. Compare this radiograph of a longitudinal stress fracture with that seen in Figure III.77.

Improvement of symptoms by rest is constant and, if there is any doubt in the diagnosis, the patient should be rested for a short while; the rapid improvement in the pain or aching will confirm the diagnosis.

TREATMENT

For the longitudinal stress fracture with severe symptoms a below-knee walking plaster is useful. In the less severe case, elastic adhesive strapping is sufficient, but with both forms of treatment activity must be kept to a level which gives rise to no symptoms. After about a month it is possible to start gradual increased activity but this must be slow and graduated or symptoms will recur. The plaster cast could be removed at three or four weeks and strapping substituted; at about six weeks all restriction can be removed but again full activity must be resumed gradually.

Transverse Stress Fractures of the Tibia

This is an extremely dangerous stress fracture which occurs in athletes or dancers, particularly those doing ballet. Initially it may not give rise to very severe symptoms but, with persistent activity, the partial stress fracture may become complete and give way with much displacement and morbidity, thus perhaps ruining a promising career.

SYMPTOMS AND SIGNS

The symptoms are very similar to any other stress fracture of the tibia with pain on activity which gradually comes on earlier during the activity and becomes persistent after the activity has finished. Rest pain occurs and, unlike other stress fractures, it is at this stage that it may fracture completely. The radiographs of such a patient are shown in Figures III.94 to III.96; he was an athlete who played American football. He was advised to stop playing. He persisted, however, and in a further game a complete fracture occurred with much displacement. It was also found that he was developing a similar fracture in the opposite leg.

The ballet dancer will notice that the pain comes on particularly when on points, or with any other steps that require much powerful flexion of the ankle and foot.

In both dancer and athlete the history can be long and spread over months rather than weeks.

The disturbance of the leg by the fracture is not very great but a small swelling can be seen on the front of the shin and, when palpated it is hard and tender (Figs. III.97 to III.99). A ballet dancer, aged 19, had had no injury and had no pain on walking. For some five months before being seen she had felt pain in the shin; this had been treated by short-wave diathermy. She then went on holiday for four weeks during which she did not dance; she got better but as soon as she returned to dancing the pain got worse. Jumping and point work were particularly noticeable as causing symptoms. Perhaps because she had had a rest during her holiday the fracture had started to heal and this is why it did not break completely with the resumption of dancing.

RADIOGRAPHY

Usually the crack, when it runs transversely across one cortex, can be seen without difficulty in the radiographs provided, as always, they are carefully centred and exposed.

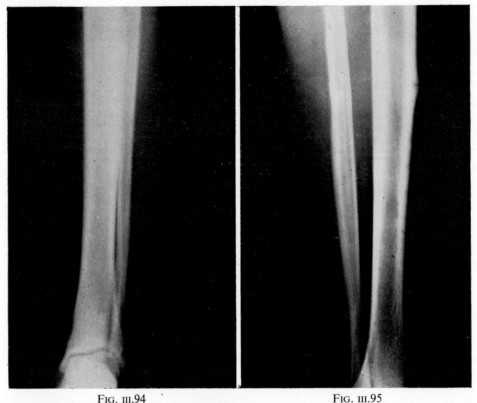

FIG. III.94   FIG. III.95

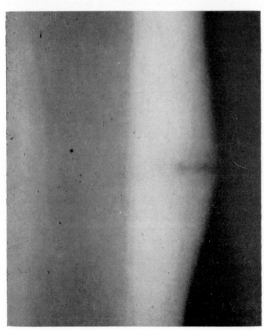

FIG. III.96

A 19-year-old man played American football. From the second game of the season he began to develop pain in his shin which was attributed to shin soreness. Rapid running or exertion caused the pain. He continued playing in spite of his symptoms. After the season was over he rested and the pain improved.

The next season he attended for advice and was found to have a transverse stress fracture. He failed to take advice and continued to play football, whereat the leg broke completely. It is interesting that the opposite leg also had a similar fracture, and it must be remembered that it is only of the worst side that the patient usually complains because the limitation of activity prevents the less severe side from hurting. Figure III.94 does not show much in the anteroposterior radiograph but in Figure III.95 the not very significant crack and the thickening of the cortex around it might mislead the unwary into thinking that the bone was safe. The enlarged view in Figure III.96 shows that the fracture is through the whole of the anterior cortex.

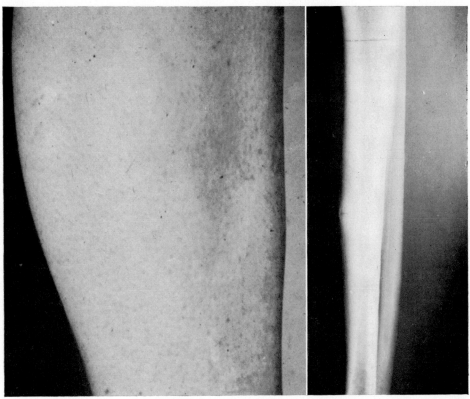

FIG. III.97   FIG. III.98

A ballet dancer aged 19 had shin soreness with no known injury. She got no pain on walking but only when she danced. During the five months history, she had been on holiday for four weeks and the pain got better but it returned when she started dancing; it was particularly painful on jumping. The clinical photograph (Fig. III.97) shows a very slight prominence on the front of the shin and the radiograph shows a small transverse fracture at this site. In both the ordinary radiograph (Fig. III.98) and in the enlarged view (Fig. III.99) the fracture does not appear to have gone right through the anterior cortex and there is a bridge of bone anteriorly, perhaps because of the four weeks rest; nevertheless this fracture is very dangerous and if the patient had continued to exercise it would have broken completely.

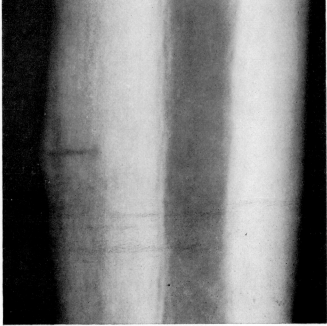

FIG. III.99

Rarely the fracture at the centre of the tibial shaft is oblique not transverse; it is not possible clinically to distinguish between the two, but radiologically it is obvious (Figs. III.100 to III.103).

At first the transverse crack, slight and seemingly innocuous, has little reaction; with continued use the lips of the fracture build up but with no evidence of union (Fig. III.96). The fracture caused by injury behaves in a very different manner, as is shown in Figures III.104 and III.105. Figure III.103 also shows how healing can be seen to be starting in a ballet dancer's tibia but, insufficiently strong after one month's rest from dancing, pain recurred.

DIAGNOSIS

It is most important to diagnose this stress fracture at once and with sufficient confidence to enable the patient to accept the treatment. Provided the condition is recognised to be hazardous, particularly in dancers and athletes, then the condition will always come to mind when pain near the centre of the shin is associated with the particular activity of the patient. Even before radiographic confirmation of the diagnosis, treatment must be started.

The activity of the patient, whether in athletics or dancing, and the general fitness entailed thereby, will eliminate most other conditions; however, tenosynovitis or the anterior tibial syndrome might be confusing to the unskilled clinician, to the danger of the patient. At the risk of seeming overanxious, if doubt about a stress fracture is present, activity must be curtailed.

If the radiographs show an oblique stress fracture at the central tibial shaft (Fig. III.100) then the same diagnosis should be maintained in regard to the treatment, since it is not known if the oblique variety at this unusual site would fracture completely and with the same ease as the true transverse type.

TREATMENT

Absolute rest from the activity causing pain must be ensured and not until the fracture has united firmly both clinically and radiologically should light training be started. The latter must be stopped should symptoms recur and a further period of rest given. Otherwise training should be continued, gradually increasing both in effort and time. It is always wise to put a plaster cast on to the athlete, either for the very precarious fracture, or for difficulty in convincing the athlete of the necessity of rest. The patient should exercise rigorously in the plaster but without too much weight-bearing.

DISCUSSION

The transverse stress fracture of the tibial shaft is uncommon when compared to the oblique shin soreness type of stress fracture; but despite that it may well cause more disability in general because it is still poorly recognised and treated too late, often only when the tibial shaft has fractured completely. Failure in diagnosis or treatment of what is, at first, a simple lesion may cause the patient to abandon a worthwhile career because of the resulting disability.

This fracture is of the type it is because of a different stress applied; perhaps this is easiest to understand in the ballet dancer doing points with intense flexion of toes, foot and ankle which will distract the anterior aspect of the tibia because of the pull

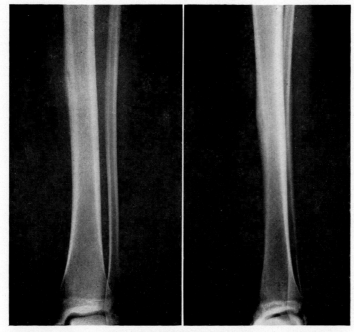

FIG. III.100   FIG. III.101

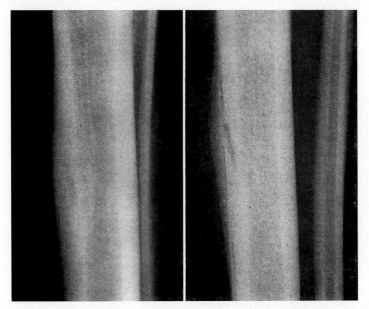

FIG. III.102   FIG. III.103

A girl of 18 was a dancer in a troupe. She developed pain in the left shin two months before being seen. The radiographs in Figures III.100 and III.101 were taken on her first visit; they show that there is a stress fracture in the centre of the tibia at the same site as the transverse stress fracture but in her particular case it is oblique and runs downwards. Perhaps the different method of dancing is the reason for the different direction of the fracture line. It should be considered just as dangerous as the transverse stress fracture until proved otherwise, but is probably much quicker to unite. Figures III.102 and III.103 are radiographs taken one month later and show union progressing.

G

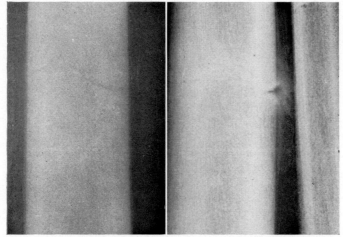

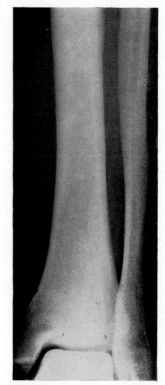

FIG. III.104   FIG. III.105

A boy of 15 had a very sharp and direct injury when his shin hit, crosswise, the shin of another player at football. He was found to have a transverse but undisplaced fracture (Fig. III.104). The radiograph taken four weeks later (Fig. III.105) shows a break in the cortex very similar to that of a transverse stress fracture but the callus outside the periosteum is quite different. However, this radiograph does show that, although the remainder of the fracture has united, part of the outer aspect of the cortex is still unhealed despite the overlying callus.

FIG. III.106

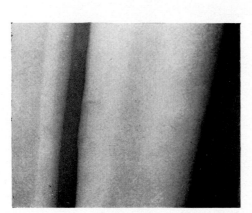

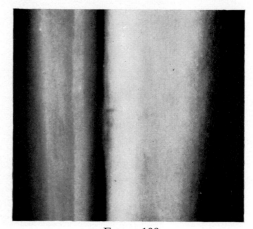

FIG. III.107   FIG. III.108

FIGS. III.106 to III.108   An international footballer developed typical shin soreness during one season. He had developed a stress fracture which can just be seen in the enlarged oblique radiograph in Figure III.107. It could not be seen in the ordinary anteroposterior radiograph (Fig. III.106). He did not play football during the summer but on the first game of the next season his leg broke in an ordinary tackle; a radiograph (Fig. III.108) shows that the fracture followed the original fracture line in Figure III.107, which can just be seen going across and a little bit upwards in the shaft of the tibia. This emphasises the importance of adequate diagnosis and treatment. He was fortunate not to have had complete displacement of the fractured tibia.

of the posterior calf muscles. The early stage of the transverse stress fracture of the tibia, when it is a thin line, is akin to the transverse stress fracture of the patella in which it is far more obvious that such a distraction must occur.

Stress Fractures of the Tibial Tubercle

In childhood the injury to the tibial tubercle called Osgood-Schlatter's disease is a stress lesion of the osteochondral junction (see Chapter Ten). The same stress may occur in young adults but, because the tibial tubercle is now firmly united to the upper epiphysis of the tibia, it becomes fractured with a greater or lesser portion of the tibial plateau breaking off with it.

SYMPTOMS AND SIGNS

The patient is usually active and youthful. Figures III.109 to III.111 show the radiographs of a boy of 16 who had had pain for two years in the region of the right knee, which he located around the tibial tubercle, always worse after energetic activity. The pain was always present after a football game. He was running, on this occasion, over flat ground, and he felt pain in his knee and fell to the ground. The history of aching for a long period is typical. The tibial tubercle has been avulsed and the fracture line extends to the tibial plateau, which is involved. The stress fracture was completely reduced and held by means of a screw. Figures III.112 to III.114 show the radiographs of a girl of 14 who was in full training for championship high jumping. Her leg gave way quite suddenly on the take-off of a jump; previously she had had pain during the season but it had not been severe. The radiographs of this girl show how the tibial tubercle has had a stress fracture through its base, and that with further stress it has broken off completely.

RADIOLOGY

The condition is not common; radiographs do not seem to have helped in diagnosis until complete separation has occurred; partly this is because the tibial tubercle, although firmly united, still has cartilage posteriorly between its tip and the upper tibia.

DIAGNOSIS

The diagnosis of a stress fracture of the tibial tubercle is based on the symptoms and signs of a stress fracture anywhere. Pain on activity which gradually gets worse, with local tenderness, should cause suspicion especially in the absence of any injury. When the pain is present with sport it is essential to consider the diagnosis. Once the fracture has been suspected careful questioning will elicit the connection with activity. Proper treatment will allow healing and thus confirm the diagnosis without the catastrophies shown in Figures III.109 to III.114.

The symptoms and signs of osteochondritis of the tibial tubercle in the younger child are well known. If a similar condition is present in a patient too old for osteochondritis there is, until proved otherwise, a developing stress fracture.

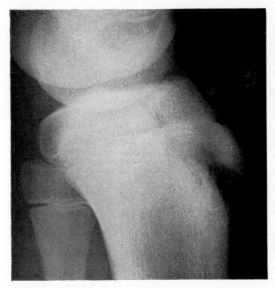

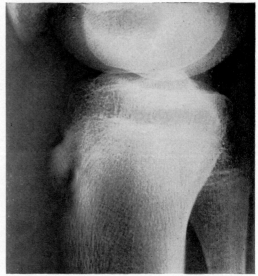

FIG. III.109

FIG. III.110

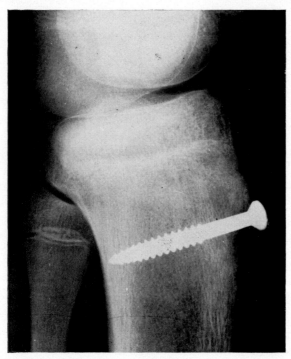

A boy of 16 had had pain for two years in the region of the right knee which he felt had been around the tibial tubercle. It was always worse after energetic activity especially after playing football. During one game, while running over flat ground, he felt a severe pain in his knee and fell to the ground. The radiograph shows that the tibial tubercle had been avulsed. The fracture line extends upwards through the still visible but united epiphysis to the tibial plateau (Fig. III.109). Figure III.110 shows the opposite knee taken at the time of admission to hospital. The fracture was reduced and fixed and he made an uneventful recovery (Fig. III.111).

FIG. III.111

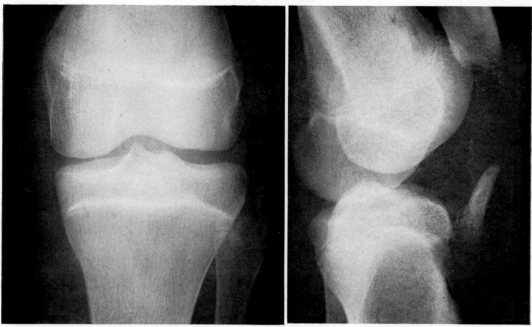

FIG. III.112	FIG. III.113

FIGS. III.112 to III.114   A girl of 14, already achieving junior championship status in sport, said that she was taking off during a high jump when her knee collapsed and she felt pain. She said that she had had pain at the same site throughout the summer but it had not been severe. The antero-posterior radiograph (Fig. III.112) would pass as normal except for the high patella. In the lateral view the severe displacement of the tibial tubercle can be seen (Fig. III.113). After open reduction and fixation with a screw (Fig. III.114) the tubercle united satisfactorily but it took many months for the patient to get back to full sport with the same efficiency as before.

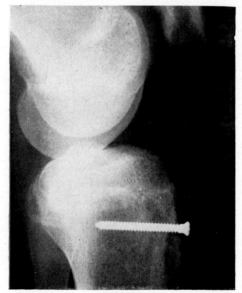

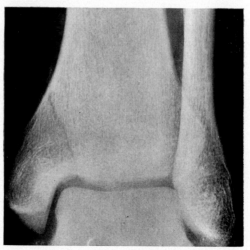

FIG. III.115

FIG. III.114

A boy of 17, keen on running, developed pain in the ankle similar to shin soreness but lower and more medially. It took three months for his stress fracture of the medial malleolus to show in this radiograph.

TREATMENT

Sport must be stopped and with it all activity likely to cause pain. Because the adolescent patient is loth either to rest or to lose time off from training, a plaster cylinder from ankle to groin for a period of two to three weeks will give a good start to healing. In the plaster, training can be continued—but the opposite knee must be examined carefully to exclude a similar but less advanced stress fracture.

Stress Fractures of the Medial Malleolus

This odd entity is real, if rare. It can occur (like any bizarre stress fracture) from an odd strain or from athletics. Figure III.115 shows the radiograph of the medial malleolus in an athlete, a boy of 17, who had a history of pain in his left big toe after training for a few days; this improved but for some reason he felt he could not bend his ankle as fully as before. However, he continued training but eight months later returned with further pain in the ankle after racing. He was found to have a swollen ankle with a tender medial malleolus; the radiograph showed a fracture line in the medial malleolus which was treated in a plaster cast. He returned to sport six weeks later.

An example of odd stress is shown in Figures III.116 to III.120. A man of 52 had an accident and broke his left tibia. The radiograph is shown in Figure III.116. The medial malleolus was intact. But he also had had an unnoticed and untreated tear of the lateral ligament of the left knee; it was only later that it was diagnosed (Fig. III.119). He obtained union of the fracture but some years later attended hospital with pain in the ankle; the pain was around the medial malleolus, which was then found to be broken with much heaped-up callus (Fig. III.118). The cause of this fracture was not appreciated until a radiograph was taken with the patient weight-bearing (Fig. III.120), which showed that most of the weight of the body was passing through the medial malleolus in which the stress fracture developed. The patient said that he had, in fact, been given a caliper but he had discarded this in favour of using one crutch and taking weight through the injured leg, despite its deformity when doing so.

The last stress fracture (Fig. III.118) is perhaps a very rare example of the transmission of weight causing the stress, instead of, as is normal, its being a stress induced by muscular pull. In the previous case of the athlete (Fig. III.115) it may well have been an abnormal style, secondary to the pain in the big toe, that altered the stress on the lower tibia so that, instead of developing shin soreness, this type of stress fracture occurred.

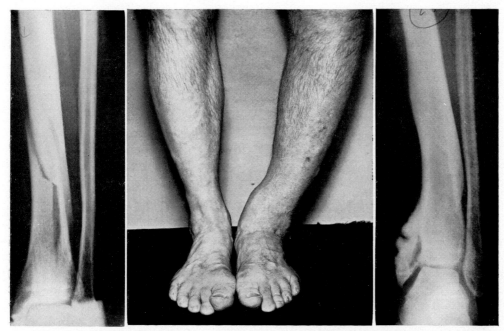

FIG. III.116   FIG. III.117   FIG. III.118

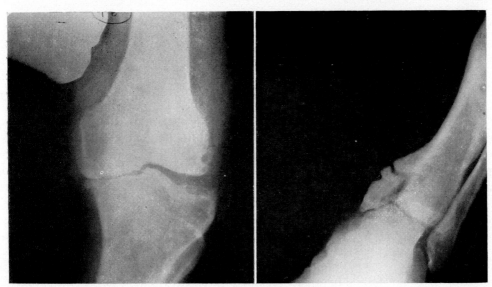

FIG. III.119   FIG. III.120

A man of 52 complained of pain in the inner side of his left ankle. Some years previously he had had a severe fracture of the tibia (Fig. III.116) and since then he said his leg had been bowed (Fig. III.117). The initial radiograph of the medial malleolus (Fig. III.118) showed a most curious condition. When strain films of the knee were taken it showed that the lateral ligament of the knee had been torn at the time of the fracture of the tibia (Fig. III.119) and a radiograph taken while weight-bearing showed that the weight passed through the medial malleolus as much as it did through the tibia (Fig. III.120). There had been no further injury. This patient had developed a stress fracture from the unaccustomed stress. Note that in the radiograph taken at the time of the accident (Fig. III.116) the medial malleolus, although not very clearly shown, certainly has not got a fracture. Full blood investigations showed no abnormality and syphilis was excluded.

CHAPTER FOUR

SIMULTANEOUS STRESS FRACTURES OF THE TIBIA AND FIBULA

About one in four stress fractures of the tibia are associated with a stress fracture of the fibula. Nine out of ten patients with this double fracture are women over the age of 60. When the condition does occur in a man there is usually in the history some predisposing cause, or possibility thereof, such as a gastrointestinal illness. The distal ends of the tibia and fibula are affected more often than the proximal ends.

At the present time idiopathic osteoporosis, particularly in older women, must be considered to be within the normal physiological expectancy of the female skeleton. The causes of osteoporosis in this sense are not known. The dividing line between what is a physiological and what is a pathological osteoporosis again is difficult to assess. Certain forms of osteoporosis are certainly induced by generalised disease, malabsorption, or by drugs. Of these, rheumatoid arthritis and steroids take pride of place partly because they so often go together. Therefore it is not surprising that women in late middle age develop stress fractures of a certain type, which although not entirely restricted to that sex, follows a very definite pattern.

SYMPTOMS AND SIGNS

In a normal woman between 60 and 70 there may be some small episode in the patient's life to which the onset of symptoms in the leg may be attributed. Thus Figure IV.1 shows the radiograph of a stress fracture in the lower tibia and fibula in a woman of 61 who had developed pain in the ankle after a move to a new flat. Sometimes the patient will think that a mild injury was the cause of the symptoms. Such a patient is shown in Figure IV.2: she said that she had strained her ankle two months previously but that there had been no bruising or other abnormality at the time. The strain that she had had was not severe but she thought the pain had persisted since then but she was unable to go into further details of the injury, which was apparently no more than the onset of pain while walking over some rough ground.

The patients will not always have pain at the ankle but they may attribute it to a worsening of arthritis of the knee. This is all the more common if the simultaneous fractures are just below the knee; the double stress fracture at this site usually occurs in the more osteoporotic patient than in the healthier or more active woman in late middle age. In general the pain is always worse with activity, but again in the older patient activity must be questioned to find out exactly what it is. This is important because the pain of a stress fracture almost invariably comes on after, and then with, activity and the duties of the older housewife or widow often involve much more work early in the day. Thus if the patient complains of pain in the middle of the day it may well be that this is after the more active hours of work. Many women tend to start the day in bedroom slippers and lack the firm support of shoes until later on, and this again may be a reason why symptoms are felt in the morning.

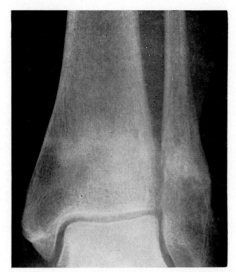

FIG. IV.1

A woman of 63 years fell in November and sustained a Colles' fracture which had united by early February the following year. She came back to hospital two weeks later complaining of pain in the left ankle. She said she had moved her flat just before the pain had started. She was treated conservatively and two months later the fractures were symptom-free. It is possible that this patient had a very mild and seronegative rheumatoid arthritis because she had a low haemoglobin content and a raised sedimentation rate.

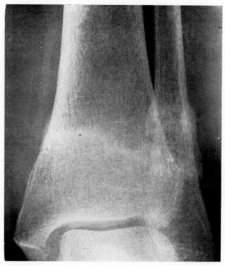

FIG. IV.2

A woman of 71 developed pain and swelling in the ankle and thought that she had strained it two months before being seen; she had noticed no bruising. She said that otherwise she was well. The radiographs here show a well-developed and uniting simultaneous stress fracture of the tibia and fibula. She made good progress with conservative treatment.

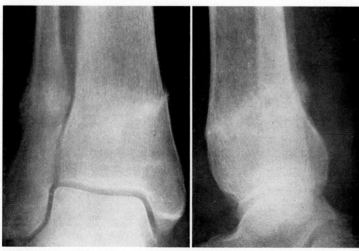

FIG. IV.3   FIG. IV.4

A woman of 61, slightly overweight, had no history of injury but had had pain and swelling of the ankle for two months. She had developed a simultaneous stress fracture of both tibia and fibula. Note that the radiographs show that there has been slight valgus angulation at the fracture site; the patient had been walking throughout and the fracture in the fibula is already uniting in these radiographs which were taken when she was first seen.

A very careful history of previous conditions must be taken to exclude any form or cause of malabsorption precipitating osteoporosis or other similar condition.

The pain slowly worsens until the patient seeks advice. With the fractures around the ankle, stability does not seem to be in any way affected, but when the fractures occur below the knee the patient can feel most unstable and is very anxious about falling. Sometimes, and much more rarely, the fractures occur in the mid-shaft of the tibia but again these are associated with the more osteoporotic patient. Occasionally there will be complaint of deformity or crookedness of the ankle, which can occur. A woman of 61 who was otherwise well and who had no history of injury developed pain and swelling of the ankle over two months; her radiographs are shown in Figures IV.3 and IV.4. When she was first seen she had a freely moving ankle but slight tenderness and a little oedema around it and above it. She walked well but the radiograph showed that the tibia and fibula had stress fractures and both showed slight angulation. They were already uniting with no treatment.

General examination will reveal a patient fit for her age; more often than not there are other conditions such as osteoarthritis or rheumatoid arthritis with or without treatment by steroids.

About half the patients will have no general abnormality with any bearing on the stress fractures and can be considered fit for their age in all respects. The leg below the knee will be swollen, painful and perhaps with a deformity which can occasionally be severe (Figs. IV.5 to IV.8). In the elderly, swelling around the ankle is not uncommon under ordinary circumstances but the stress fracture above the ankle will cause very considerable oedema. If the fractures are just below the knee the swelling may encompass the whole of the lower leg and appear to involve the knee itself, though there will be no fluid in the joint. Tenderness will be found all round the site of the fractures, but may be more intense on one side or the other. Because the tenderness has been found at the upper or lower part of the leg it does not mean that the rest of that part will be free of trouble, as is shown in Figures IV.5 to IV.8.

Deformity in itself may predispose to this fracture as it sometimes does in other stress fractures. Figure IV.9 shows the radiograph of a woman of 69 who had severe osteoarthritis of the left knee which for eight to ten weeks had necessitated crutches to relieve pain. Some ten months after this episode, pain occurred in the lower end of the left tibia which was at first attributed to a wasp sting by the patient and to gout by the doctor. There was redness and swelling at the time, she said, but no injury. The radiographs show not only the simultaneous stress fracture of both lower tibia and fibula but also that the fibula appears to have a more advanced fracture than the tibia; both fractures are very like those that occur singly in patients of the same age. Although that part of the double fracture in the tibia does not appear to have involved the medial cortex, there is some callus on the medial border of the tibia to be seen in the radiograph.

RADIOLOGY

Although the symptoms are often severe at the start, it is usual for the radiographs to show nothing for the first few weeks and sometimes months. The fibula shows the lesion first, as is well illustrated in Figures IV.10 and IV.11; the patient, a woman of 62, had complained of pain in the lateral side of the ankle but hardly mentioned pain on the medial side. The initial radiograph (Fig. IV.10) shows a typical stress fracture of

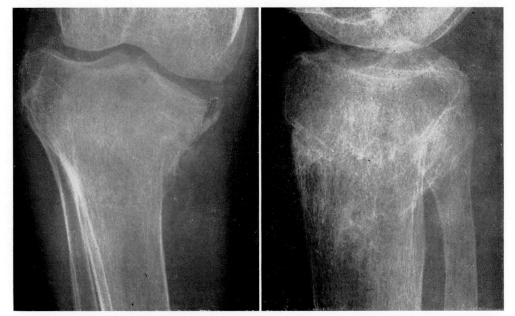

FIG. IV.5   FIG. IV.6

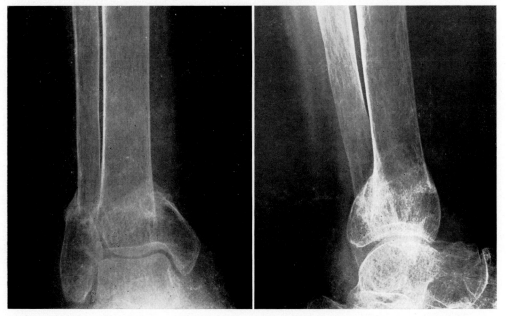

FIG. IV.7   FIG. IV.8

A woman of 72 was thought to have a malabsorption syndrome and was being investigated for this as an in-patient when she developed pain in the leg. She had developed simultaneous stress fractures of the tibia and fibula at its lower end and also of the tibia at its upper end; the fibula was also thought to have a stress fracture at its upper end but the radiographs were never very clear.

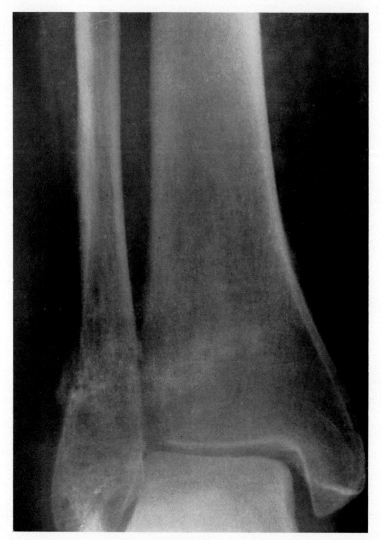

FIG. IV.9

A woman of 69 had severe osteoarthritis of the left knee which necessitated the use of crutches for eight to ten weeks. About ten months after this she developed pain in the lower end of the left tibia which she thought might have been the result of a wasp sting but which her doctor thought was gout. There was redness and swelling. There was no history of injury. The ankle remained painful on weight-bearing. The radiograph shows a simultaneous stress fracture of the lower tibia and fibula with slight valgus angulation of the lower fragment of the fibula. The well-developed fibula stress fracture shows the start of union but the tibia appears to have lagged behind, although callus is present on its medial cortex. She did well, despite being overweight, with conservative treatment.

the fibula; however, six weeks later the fracture in the lower part of the tibia was visible (Fig. IV.11). Two months later all symptoms had resolved. The radiological progress of the simultaneous fractures follows this pattern of fibula involvement being seen first and even healing before the tibial stress fracture is seen. Union of the fibula can be solid with loss of symptoms from the lateral side of the ankle while the tibia continues to give pain. Such a patient is shown in Figure IV.12—a woman who was on steroids after having a carcinoma of the breast removed. She complained of pain in the ankle and a stress fracture of the fibula was diagnosed and began to heal satisfactorily, but, to the surprise of the clinician, the pain in the ankle continued and further radiography showed the development of the compression stress fracture in the lower end of the tibia. The radiograph of this patient also shows that the simultaneous stress fractures are not always at exactly the same level; here the fibula has had a fracture some distance above the lateral malleolus but the tibial fracture was low down. Sometimes both the stress fractures will be high above the ankle, as is shown in the radiograph in Figure IV.13 of a patient who was only 64 and who had had rheumatoid arthritis treated by steroids for many years. She had also had hydrocortisone injections into her knees on many occasions and she had worn a caliper on the right lower leg. One day the leg began to ache; a little while later she decided to try managing without the caliper but the pain became worse. Not only had she developed a stress fracture at the junction of the middle and lowest thirds of the tibia and fibula but there was also a second double fracture very low down and only just above the ankle. The upper fractures show deformity but she made an uninterrupted recovery with simple conservative methods.

The swelling of the leg may mask the deformity that is found radiologically. Figures IV.14 and IV.15 show the radiographs of a patient of 78 who had to be admitted to hospital as an emergency because of the pain in her leg. Her history was that she had had cramp in the left calf some weeks before which had made her limp and she had had pain up the left leg. The swelling of the ankle hid the deformity which is clearly shown in the radiograph, and which needed manipulation under an anaesthetic before a plaster cast was applied in which the fracture united with no further trouble. This patient had without doubt some osteoporosis, but not to an unusual amount for her age.

Radiography may also show stress fractures in the elderly when none is suspected clinically. Such was the case in a woman of 90 who was admitted from a nursing home to a geriatric unit for rehabilitation because she had 'gone off her feet'. There was no history of any injury. She complained of some pain in the knee and the radiograph showed a stress fracture of the tibia and fibula just below the knee (Fig. IV.16). She developed bronchopneumonia and died. She had had both her hips treated for fractures many years previously. Again, one double stress fracture may mask the symptoms from another. The patient whose radiographs are shown in Figures IV.5 to IV.8 had a malabsorption syndrome and was in hospital being investigated for this when she developed pain in the leg. Not only had she got a simultaneous stress fracture of the tibia and fibula at its lower end but also in the upper part, which was not suspected clinically. This patient had osteoporosis in which condition stress fractures are very common but not always recognised as such.

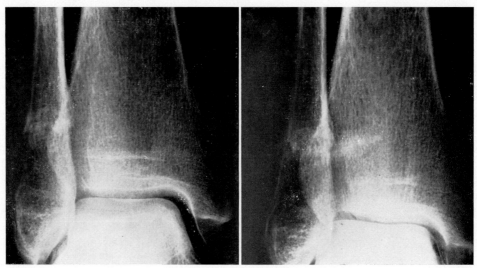

FIG. IV.10   FIG. IV.11

A woman of 62 had had pain for six weeks in the lateral side of her right ankle. This was diagnosed as a stress fracture of the fibula but a further radiograph six weeks later showed that the tibia was also involved. She was free of symptoms in a further two months.

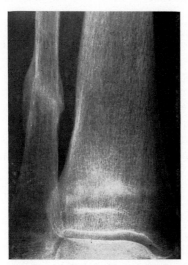

FIG. IV.12

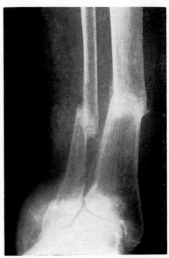

FIG. IV.13

A woman of 64 who had been on steroids for 18 months after a carcinoma of the breast developed a stress fracture of the fibula. She was also rather more tender than usual around the lower end of the tibia and it was thought possible that the tibia had also a stress fracture. This showed three months later when this radiograph was taken. Later on, having had a successful knee replacement on the left side, she developed a stress fracture of the neck of the left femur, probably because the painful knee had prevented her from much walking before the arthroplasty.

A woman of 64 had rheumatoid arthritis treated by steroids over many years. She had also had hydrocortisone injections to her knees on many occasions and had worn a caliper on the right lower leg. One day she got out of bed without a caliper because her leg had been aching the day previously and she thought it might be better without the iron. The pain became severe and she attended hospital where the simultaneous stress fractures at two levels were found. She made a good recovery in 14 weeks. The lower fractures are very close to the ankle.

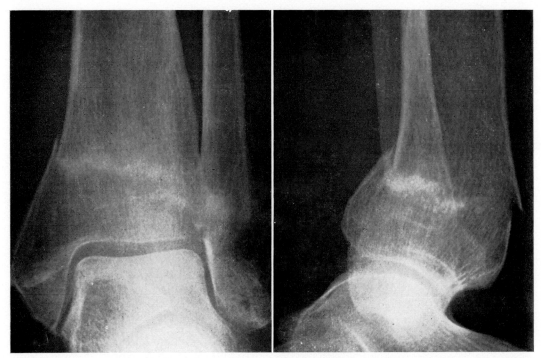

FIG. IV.14 FIG. IV.15

FIG. IV.14 FIG. IV.15

A woman of 78 was admitted as an emergency. She said that she had had cramp in the left calf some weeks before which had caused her to walk with a limp and she had had pain up the left leg. She was found to have a stress fracture of the tibia and fibula which needed manipulation under anaesthetic. She was then put into a below-knee plaster on which she was able to walk. The displacement must have increased shortly before her admission and caused the increased pain, but the fracture had been present for some weeks.

FIG. IV.16

A woman of 90 had had bilateral fractures of the femur previously and had been in a nursing home. There was no history of a fall and it was most unlikely that she had had an injury. She was admitted to a geriatric unit for rehabilitation, and the stress fracture of the tibia and fibula was discovered incidentally when she complained of pain in the knee while she was having treatment for a pressure sore on the heel. She developed bronchopneumonia later and died.

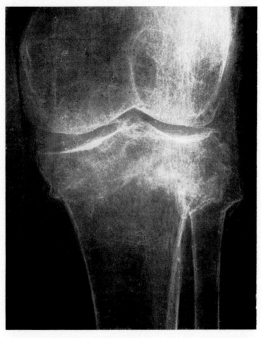

FIG. IV.16

DIAGNOSIS

Osteoporotic bones may be tender. In the decades between 60 and 90 there are many other conditions which cause a general tenderness of the bones. However, any localised tenderness, whatever the general condition of the patient, with swelling, redness and a history of pain on activity must cause the suspicion of a stress fracture and this can usually be confirmed radiologically although it must be remembered that some of the fractures take a considerable time to show radiologically.

The main conditions which may be confused with stress fractures of the type under consideration and in the group concerned are arthritis, either primary or secondary, vascular disease, varicose veins and varicose ulcers, systemic conditions that can be localised to a part, such as gout; occasionally a secondary neoplasm, which can occur in the tibia, may have to be considered. All general conditions, such as myelomatosis, must be excluded by routine investigations even if the stress fracture has been diagnosed as such. Malabsorption syndromes and other pathological causes of osteoporosis must be excluded.

DISCUSSION

The stress fractures that occur simultaneously in the tibia and fibula are undoubtedly an indication of weakening of the bones with ageing. It must be accepted that, with our present inadequate knowledge, osteoporosis is a usual concomitant of old age, especially in women, in whom these stress fractures are very much more often found than they are in men. Osteoporosis varies from person to person, each of whom can otherwise be normal for their age. In the same way that the child develops a compression stress fracture of the tibia, and interestingly enough in its uppermost third where some of the older patients also develop this stress fracture, so the bone of childhood is different from that of the healthy adult. But the bone of a child is growing and has to accept the ever-increasing muscle strength and to withstand the everyday activities of the child. In the same way the bone of the older person loses unnecessary strength because the muscle tone decreases even under ordinary circumstances of good general health. Bone is unable to maintain strength without the stimulus of the stress of muscle tone that is placed upon it. Immobilisation lowers muscle tone; the bones immobilised also become weaker and osteoporotic. In the older person muscle tone decreases as does the strength of the muscles. Until we have discovered how to prevent the loss of strength, and tone, in muscles as age increases, osteoporosis will continue and with it a decreased strength of the bone and inability to withstand stress.

Because women do get more and more osteoporotic they will sustain very severe stress fractures which may be a terminal event. An extreme example is shown in Figures IV.17 to IV.19, which illustrate the lower leg of a woman of 83. She was somewhat senile and had developed simultaneous stress fractures of the tibia and fibula, just above the ankle, which were present for some considerable time. In an attempt to preserve her well-being she was put into a walking plaster but she fell and broke her hip and had to be admitted to hospital, when she died. Figures IV.17 and IV.18 show the radiographs of the stress fracture, and Figure IV.19 is a photograph of the specimen taken with ultraviolet light. The patient had been on tetracycline previously, and the fluorescence seen in the lower tibia indicates that new bone formation has been going on for some considerable time.

In this chapter all the patients described had osteoporosis to a greater or lesser

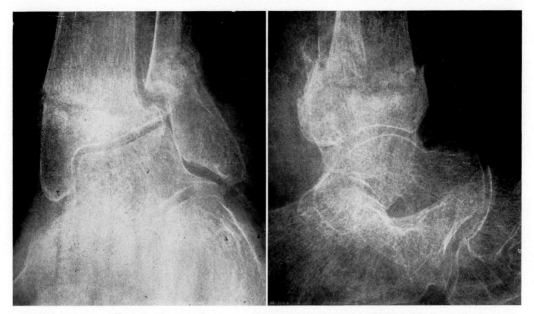

FIG. IV.17   FIG. IV.18

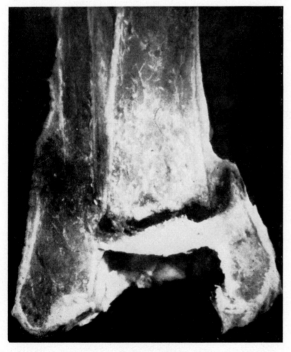

FIG. IV.19

A senile woman of 83 developed a painful swollen left foot and ankle with no history of injury. She was found to have a stress fracture of both the lower tibia and fibula (Figs. IV.17 and IV.18). She was allowed to walk in a plaster cast but she fell and was admitted to hospital having fractured her left hip, and despite treatment she did not survive. The patient also had diabetes. She had been on tetracycline previously and the photograph of the specimen in Figure IV.19 taken under fluorescent light shows the new bone formation.

H

degree. It is still considered that the stress fractures that occurred fulfil to a sufficient extent the criteria of occurring in the normal bone of a normal person because it is normal to find osteoporosis in the elderly, and age in itself cannot be ascribed to abnormality. The dividing line between the mature strong bone of the young athlete and that of an active 80-year-old is tenuous and, although at each extreme the difference is obvious, year by year the change must progress, so that in any one person it is impossible to say that at a specific time the bone has become abnormal.

CHAPTER FIVE

STRESS FRACTURES OF THE FEMUR

Stress fractures of the femur divide themselves into two main groups, those of the shaft and those of the upper end near the hip. The most common site is the femoral neck, which sustains stress fractures at all ages and in both sexes but in the older patient there is a heavy predominance in women. In the latter group of patients there is no doubt that osteoporosis has a greater or lesser part to play in the same way that it does in the compression stress fracture of the tibia, as has been seen in Chapters Three and Four. Deep x-ray therapy to the pelvis has in the past been a cause of weakening of the bones in that area and may predispose to a form of stress fracture in the femoral neck. However, many stress fractures of the femoral neck are seen in healthy fit young adults and if not recognised and treated correctly may be a disaster to the patient, who remains disabled for life.

The much less common stress fracture of the shaft of the femur is seen at all ages but also in the healthy young adult, in whom it occurs in men probably because it is associated with heavy or arduous exercise although there is no reason to suppose that a young woman taking similar activity should not also get this fracture.

One interesting and important point about stress fractures of the femur is that they are very commonly bilateral, whether in the femoral shaft or in the femoral neck, and this must never be forgotten when treating a patient with this condition.

Stress Fractures of the Femoral Shaft

The femoral shaft sustains a transverse or longitudinal stress fracture with no abnormal, though often unusual, activity. An excellent example of this is shown in the radiographs of the femur of an 18-year-old marine who had been in the service for nine months (Figs. v.1 to v.3). He fell somewhat awkwardly from a height of 4 feet which, for a marine commando, is trivial, but his femur was broken (Fig. v.3). Routine radiography of the opposite femur to measure the length of the Küntscher nail that was to be used showed there was a stress fracture in that bone as well, which is shown in Figures v.1 and v.2. There was no history of symptoms from either femur, nor had he any unusual deformities or accidents and he was entirely fit at the time. This type of fracture is transverse, like that which occurs in the tibia, and, as can readily be appreciated, it will break across the second cortex with disastrous results. Close inspection of the radiograph in Figure v.3 shows that the cortex on the lateral side is thickened, both on its superficial and deep surfaces, and matches very closely the pattern of the stress fracture seen in Figure v.2, which might well have broken instead. There can be no doubt that both femora had stress fractures and that the trivial injury was sufficient to break the opposite cortex from the side of the stress fracture. It must be remembered that bilateral stress fractures are common and always to be expected.

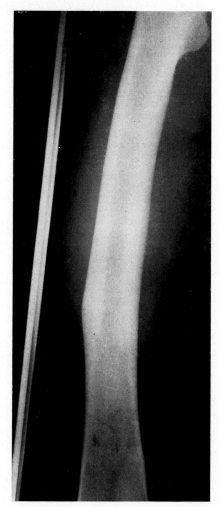

FIG. v.I

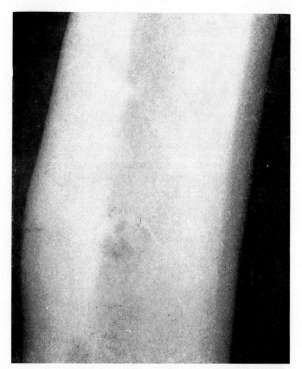

FIG. v.2

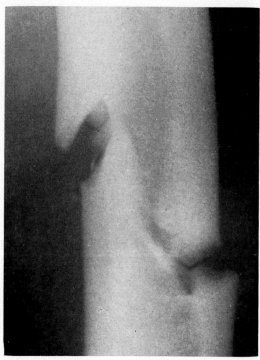

FIG. v.3

A marine commando aged 18 had completed nine months in the service when he had a trivial fall but found that his leg was broken. Routine radiography of the opposite femoral shaft to determine the length of the Küntscher nail that should be used revealed a stress fracture in the outer cortex of that bone about the centre of the shaft (Fig. v.1). This fracture is shown better in the enlarged view in Figure v.2. It will be seen that the stress fracture runs transversely through the lateral cortex, which is much thickened. When the fracture of the opposite femur is looked at closely in the enlarged view it can be seen that the cortex has also become thickened on its lateral aspect. There can be no doubt that this fracture, shown in Figure v.3, was a complication of a pre-existing transverse fracture in the outer cortex of the femur.

SYMPTOMS AND SIGNS

The lack of symptoms in a stress fracture of the femur can mislead. It is unusual to have a very long history of severe pain.

This absence of severe symptoms must not detract from making the diagnosis, especially when a patient attends with a mild aching in the thigh over a period of weeks, or even with the complaint of muscular stiffness in the region of the hip or knee. It may only occur with exercise such as running or on long marches and, as with other stress fractures, it disappears with rest. There will be no history of injury, and there is unlikely to be any history of any other condition having any bearing on the stress fracture apart, of course, from the activity of the patient, which must be gone into with great care, as is shown by the history of the patient illustrated in Figures v.4 to v.6. The patient, on first attending, may walk with a limp, but although there is complaint of pain and stiffness of knee or hip gentle examination will show no limitation of movement. There will be local tenderness in the thigh at the site of the fracture varying with the degree to which it has progressed. Rotation of the femur against resistance, done by holding the lower leg with the knee bent and rotating it medially or laterally, may produce the pain, as may forced abduction or adduction. It is wise not to be too forceful with these manoeuvres when a transverse stress fracture is suspected in the femur, or for that matter in any other bone. Some wasting may be apparent in the quadriceps or calf muscles.

RADIOLOGY

The femur, like the tibia, can fracture transversely or longitudinally. Figures v.1 to v.3 show the bilateral transverse stress fractures; Figures v.4 to v.6 show the longitudinal fracture which, because it had never been seen before, needed biopsy to establish the diagnosis. They also show the difficulty of assessing the longitudinal stress fracture of the femoral shaft; never should there be hesitation before—or remorse after—doing a biopsy if the diagnosis is in doubt; in the radiograph in the anteroposterior plane the longitudinal crack passing to the lateral cortex can be seen low down and a short distance above the lateral condyle. The fracture extends well up the shaft of the femur.

Figures v.7 to v.9 show a transverse fracture in the shaft of a femur which is osteoporotic and more bowed than usual, perhaps from mild childhood rickets. It is similar to those transverse stress fractures that occur in the centre shaft of the tibia. That the stress fracture has been present for some while is shown by the thickening of the femoral cortex through which the fracture runs.

Both the transverse and the longitudinal fractures may be deceptive radiologically. The earliest sign of the transverse crack may be a little thickening both on the inside and outside of the lateral cortex, which may be all that can be discerned unless the fine fracture line is shown by the x-ray beam aligned to pass perpendicularly through the fracture. The same will apply to the longitudinal crack, as in the tibia.

DIAGNOSIS

This can be difficult but the diagnosis can be made on the clinical history of pain related to activity and the results of a careful examination which will elicit tenderness. So often is pain in the hip referred to the thigh that the radiograph may have been taken of the femoral neck and upper femoral shaft only, in which case the diagnosis will not be confirmed radiologically and a disaster may occur by the fracture becoming complete.

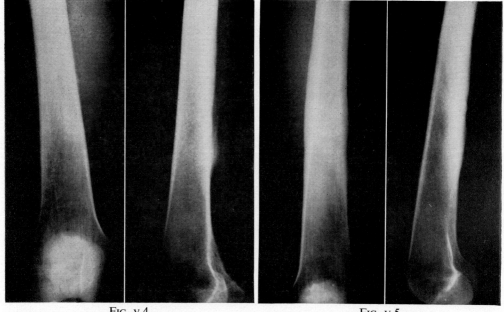

FIG. V.4   FIG. V.5

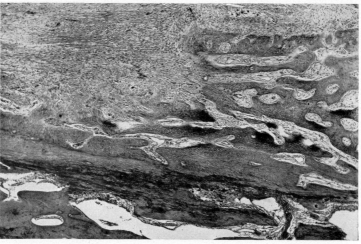

FIG. V.6

A 35-year-old office worker developed a painful stiffness of the left knee and hip. He had had no accident. Close enquiry revealed that it was his habit to run for his train every morning and that it was after this that the aching first started. He also said he had pain in the top of the knee if he ran. He had slight tenderness just above this area and the radiograph showed a longitudinal stress fracture (Fig. v.4). This was not recognised at the time, and a tumour was suspected and a biopsy was done. During his recovery from the latter the fracture healed. Figure v.5 is a radiograph of the femur one year later when the patient was entirely free of symptoms. The biopsy showed fibrous tissue with areas of regular new bone formation (Fig. v.6). There was no evidence of infection or malignancy. The appearance is that of normal fracture healing.

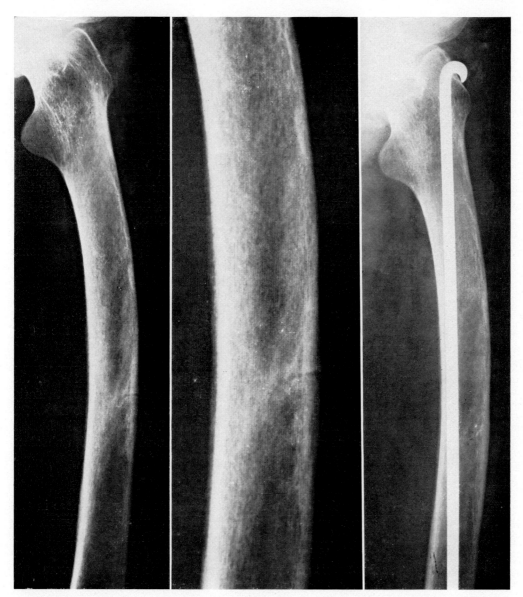

FIG. V.7   FIG. V.8   FIG. V.9

A 58-year-old maid, who worked in a hospital, began to get aching in the thigh. The radiograph showed osteoporosis and a fracture line in the outer cortex of the centre of the femoral shaft. Full investigation did not reveal any cause for the osteoporosis nor did she have any osteomalacia. She was treated by internal fixation with a Rush pin and she made a rapid recovery. It is interesting that some years later the patient developed a similar stress fracture in the opposite femur. She declined a second operation and the fracture healed with restriction of weight-bearing and activity.

Clinical examination will have shown the full range of movement of hip and knee and will have found the localised tenderness. The proper radiography will confirm the lesion.

The awareness of the condition occurring in young adults in particular or in the osteoporotic or bowed femoral shaft in the older patient will bring the diagnosis to mind as soon as the history relating pain with exercise has been given.

Any real doubt about a tumour being the cause of the pain, especially in the longitudinal variety in which the subperiosteal new bone formation may simulate a new growth, should be dispelled by the histology of the material obtained at biopsy. All forms of malabsorption and osteoporosis must be considered as a predisposing cause in the older patient, but the young adult is always found to be healthy. In the older patient the symptoms may suggest intermittent claudication although the unusually high situation in the thigh, and the timing of the pain, does not follow accurately that of vascular insufficiency. Referred pain from the low back or true sciatic pain can be distinguished by the local tenderness in the thigh and absence of any neurological signs.

The thickened cortex might, radiologically, inspire the diagnosis of an osteoid osteoma which, when looked for, will not be found.

TREATMENT

For the transverse stress fracture in a young adult, internal fixation with a suitable pin is the quickest and easiest way of ensuring the healing of the bone and the safety of the patient. A heavy intramedullary nail is not necessary because the stress fracture is caused by only a slight overload and the simpler fixation with a thin pin will redress the balance of stress. In the bilateral fracture, if one side has broken completely the rest entailed by the operation will be sufficient to allow the other side to heal, particularly if the patient is not hurried on to crutches, on which it is important not to allow the patient until making sure that the opposite femur is normal. In a longitudinal stress fracture up the shaft of the femur conservative measures are sufficient with absolute rest from all activities that cause the pain.

DISCUSSION

Stress fractures in the femoral shaft are very uncommon compared to those in the tibia. They occur either as a transverse or a longitudinal fracture. Compression and oblique stress fractures have not been seen in the femoral shaft although there is no reason to suppose that they should not occur above the femoral condyle.

Prevention of a stress fracture is always difficult but perhaps in military recruits it is easier than in other situations. The young serviceman soon develops his musculature but the bone strength, whether of the femur, tibia or metatarsal bones, does not increase so rapidly. Therefore gradual training without too energetic jumping or route marching at first will allow time for the bone to strengthen. It is impossible to repeat too often that a bone is only as strong as it needs to be, and takes time to become stronger, and that this time is never as quick as that to develop the muscles. Furthermore, most recruits put on weight with service conditions of exercise and adequate diet which indirectly increases the muscular stresses on various bones which need yet more time to strengthen.

The importance of the stress fracture of the shaft of the femur is in its danger to the patient in whom complete fracture with displacement may occur and the ease with which this can be prevented if it is diagnosed in time.

Stress Fractures of the Neck of the Femur

These are divisible into two, those that are basically distracted, or being pulled open (Fig. v.10) and those that are compressed (Fig. v.11). Stress fractures of the femoral neck are found in all age groups from the young adult onwards. They are not seen in the femoral neck of the child or adolescent until the upper femoral epiphysis is closed.

The young service recruit and the athlete are at risk of a fractured neck of femur and, if the symptoms are not recognised, catastrophies can occur because of a complete fracture with displacement. In the older patient it is wise to use internal fixation in all patients unless there are strong grounds for not operating. In patients with the distraction stress fracture immediate internal fixation or replacement is needed.

Stress Fractures of the Femoral Neck in Young and Middle-aged Adults

In the young adult a stress fracture of the femoral neck occurs with a strenuous way of life (Figs. v.10 and v.11). They do not seem to occur so commonly in athletes as they do with the heavier activities of military service, particularly in those training on first joining the service.

Symptoms and Signs

The patient may attend after the hip has given way (Figures v.12 and v.13). Careful enquiry may reveal little or no evidence of pre-existing pain in the hip. On other occasions the patient will say that there had been a gradual aching in the hip which has got worse with activity and which would then improve with rest or a few days leave. Pain after particularly severe exercise may become so bad that the activity has to be stopped. Sometimes sport can be inculpated, as with the girl in Figures v.14 to v.16 who was particularly keen on tennis. Careful enquiry must always be made for a history of pain on the opposite side, even though it is rare for it to be found, despite the fact that often such fractures are bilateral, as in this particular tennis player. This is because the symptoms on the worst side prevent activity being sufficient to allow the lesser stress fracture to develop fully on the opposite side and to cause pain. The slight haze of internal new bone can just be seen in the 'normal' hip in Figure v.15.

There is no clear-cut distinction between the various ages at which a stress fracture of the femoral neck occurs except that in the young and old disaster can supervene while those aged from about 30 to 50 years have far less chance of a displaced fracture and, in many, there is or has been some other condition that may have enhanced the possibility of a stress fracture.

Radiology

The correct understanding of the radiology of stress fractures of the femoral neck is very important because on this interpretation will depend the urgent necessity of treatment or otherwise. In Figure v.11 is seen a healing compression stress fracture of the undersurface of the neck of the femur in a soldier who was aged 20 and although the symptoms may be quite severe with this fracture it is unlikely to cause difficulty

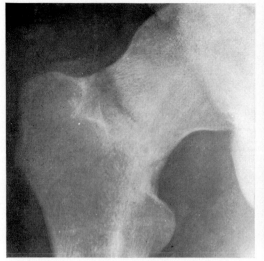

FIG. v.10

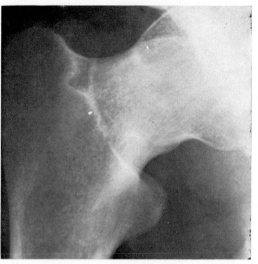

FIG. v.11

A soldier, 20 years of age, developed pain in the right hip which gradually became worse; after running five miles he was unable to walk on it. Examination showed limitation of right hip movement, and the radiograph shows clearly a distraction stress fracture in the upper surface of the neck of the femur which can also be seen going right through the lower cortex which is cracked. Without proper treatment this fracture will become as badly displaced as that in Figures v.12 and v.13.

A soldier of 20 had pain in his right hip after some strenuous work. He has developed a stress fracture of the neck of the left femur but this was in its lowest aspect only, through the inferior cortex, and was compression in type. It is already healing at the time of the first radiograph shown here. There is little danger of severe displacement in this type, particularly when compared to those shown in the preceding and following radiographs.

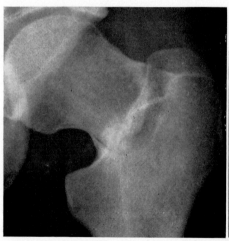

FIG. v.12

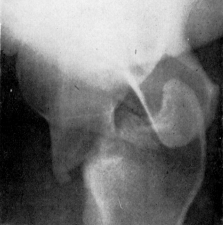

FIG. v.13

A marine of 30 collapsed some two or three miles from the end of a 30-mile speed march. He said his left hip had given way. He was unable to walk and was found to have had a fracture of the neck of the femur. There had been no injury. The radiograph shows a displaced stress fracture of the neck of the femur which follows a fairly similar pattern to that shown in Figure v.10. The hip was reduced with great difficulty and pinned. Once displaced, these fractures have a poor prognosis and often leave the patient with considerable disability.

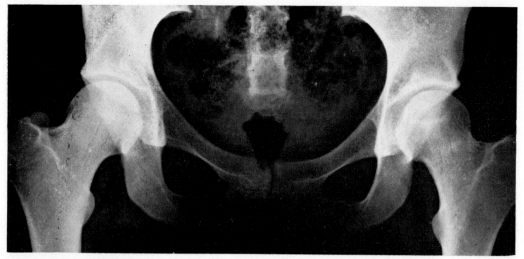

FIG. v.14

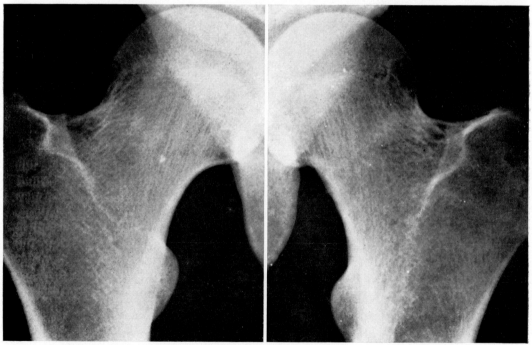

FIG. v.15   FIG. v.16

A girl of 19 who was a very keen tennis player developed pain in the left hip which started some two hours after exercise and which gradually got worse. It had been present for four weeks when she attended for advice and she was treated by non-weight-bearing of the affected leg. This was dangerous without careful assessment of the opposite leg, which in fact had an early stress fracture more easily seen in the original radiograph than in the reproduction. The fracture in Figure v.14 is quite easily seen, with a small break in the inferior cortex, and better seen in Figure v.16. In Figure v.15 there is a faint haze of new bone, as internal callus, in the neck of the right femur which fortunately did not develop further even with the excess exercise. The haze of internal callus in the femoral neck is comparable to that seen in the tibia in compression stress fractures and will be referred to later under femoral head stress fractures.

in treatment. Conversely, the distraction variety is liable to severe displacement and must be treated as a surgical emergency. The type of stress fracture shown in Figure v.10 is a good example of the dangerous variety that must be treated at once because it is liable to displacement, as is shown in Figures v.12 and v.13.

The very small amount of internal callus that may be seen is shown well in Figures v.14 to v.16. The very slight external callus on the undersurface of the neck of the left femur should be noted; also the right hip, about which there was no complaint, shows a much earlier stage of a similar stress fracture. Search must always be made for bilateral lesions.

Not all stress fractures are as obvious as that in Figure v.17, a woman of 40 who perhaps had a mild malabsorption syndrome after a gastrectomy five years previously. This is the typical compression stress fracture with a crack in the bottom cortex of the base of the femoral neck and much internal callus.

The difficulty of radiological diagnosis is illustrated in Figure v.18 which is the tomograph of the left femoral neck of a girl of 24. The fracture had not been diagnosed on routine radiography—although it was possible to do so had the signs been appreciated—until the tomograph was taken and the internal callus and the fracture line through the inferior cortex were recognised; by then, being three months after the onset of symptoms, healing was almost complete.

Continued use despite pain in the ordinary patient may cause odd radiological appearances, as is shown in the radiographs of a woman of 36 who thought she had cramp (Figs. v.19 and v.20). The fracture has continued to advance at one place and to heal at another, to give the particularly curious pattern in the left femoral neck shown in Figure v.20 while the right hip shows a more usual pattern in the radiograph in Figure v.19.

Stress Fractures of the Femoral Neck in the Older Patient

Although stress fractures of the femoral neck occur through life, from the young adult onwards, they become more common after the age of 60. Some of the patients in whom they occur between the ages of 30 and 60 have some generalised disease which may affect the strength of the bone, such as rheumatoid arthritis, treated with or without steroids, or malabsorption syndromes. In the very old patient, unless the history is carefully taken, it may well be considered that the fracture of the neck of the femur was caused by a fall at home. Below the age of 60 about half the fractures are of the compression variety and the other half distraction, but over the age of 60 they are almost invariably the distraction type that will inevitably proceed to a complete fracture and severe deformity.

SYMPTOMS AND SIGNS

These will vary with the age and activity of the patient but in general the patient complains of a dull ache in the hip region, which is often put down to rheumatism or osteoarthritis. The pain, as in the younger patient, may be referred from the hip to the knee or down the thigh. Exercise will cause the ache but, in the old person, the amount of activity in general is not always sufficiently great for the patient to realise that it is exercise in fact that is making the pain worse. Rest pain may occur and sometimes even the weight of the bedclothes on the foot may cause pain in the hip

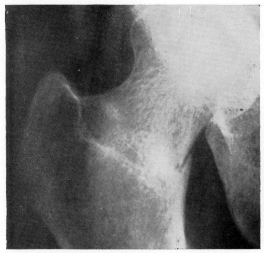

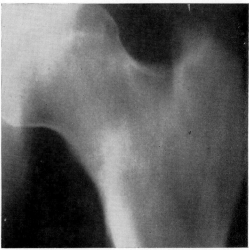

FIG. v.17

FIG. v.18

A woman of 40 years had had a gastrectomy for duodenal ulcer five years previously. Her complaint was pain in the right groin which had been present for one month. The initial radiograph showed a more than usually extensive compression stress fracture which appears to have shortened slightly even though it is difficult to see that the fracture is complete. Three weeks later radiographs showed that the fracture was beginning to unite. She had had a stress fracture of the fibula on the opposite side a year previously.

An extremely overweight girl of 24 complained of a severe pain in the left hip. Over the next three months the patient was investigated until tomography revealed a healing stress fracture, which is shown in the figure. The fracture line can still be seen at the base of the femoral neck in this figure, but the upper part of the neck appears to be normal. Internal callus surrounds the fracture line and the undersurface of the neck shows the smooth outline of a little external callus, indicating satisfactory healing.

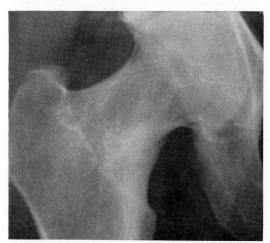

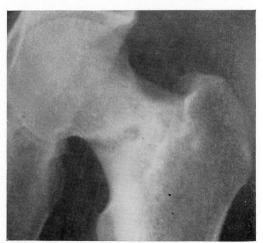

FIG. v.19

FIG. v.20

A woman of 36 years had pain in both thighs which was first felt as a cramp in the right thigh after she had sat in a cinema. She attended two weeks later as an out-patient, and the initial radiograph of the right hip (Fig. v.19) showed a compression stress fracture. The opposite hip (Fig. v.20) also had a stress fracture but of not quite the same appearance. At that time the condition was not recognised for what it was, so after a month of intensive investigations, all of which were normal, the right hip was treated by a Smith-Petersen nail. It healed very satisfactorily and while that occurred the left hip also healed with the rest that was given after the operation.

and make resting at night difficult. The fit patient may have a history of more than a month of aching and pain which may not be severe enough to necessitate advice until, perhaps, some trivial injury or stumble exacerbates the pain (Figs. v.21 and v.22).

In the very old, the history is often that of a fall at home with such an obvious fracture of the neck of the femur that the patient is thought to have had an accident. In many patients thus admitted to hospital careful enquiry in the peace and calm after the operation has been done, and when the patient is no longer anxious, frightened or confused, will reveal that for some weeks or even months there had been pain in the hip and that this had preceded the so-called fall; the patient may remember that while standing still or walking across a flat surface the hip 'gave way' with pain felt before hitting the floor. The fact that the patient with a fractured neck of femur that has broken completely and has displaced feels the pain before actually reaching the ground is diagnostic of this condition but at this stage, of course, it is too late for measures to be taken to prevent the displacement.

According to the severity of the stress fracture so will the signs of a fracture be present, with hip movements limited in most directions, or, if the fracture is complete and has displaced, the findings will be those of a fracture of the neck of the femur. Distraction stress fractures may produce considerable pain and distress within a very short time but compression stress fractures of the neck of the femur are usually less severe and less rapid in developing signs; occasionally these are seen over the age of 60. Figures v.23 and v.24 show the radiographs of a woman of 68 who had had pain in both hips for some three weeks. She had two falls after the pain had started but the radiographs show the quite typical pattern of the compression stress fracture of the base of the neck on its inferior cortical surface, even though she was older than usual for this type of fracture. She did well and obtained full movements in both hips and sound union with rest for three weeks followed by carefully guarded walking. Around the fracture at the base of the neck the sclerosed bone indicates that the fracture has been present for some time and the fracture line, being so obvious, also indicates that movement still occurs at the fracture—keeping it open and preventing union—and that rest or internal fixation is still needed.

In the patient who has been developing pain very slowly over many weeks or months physical signs may be almost entirely absent and the fracture only found on radiography. Sometimes pain is felt in both thighs which is often attributed to rheumatism or 'cramp' caused by sitting in a draught or some other similar hazard of the elderly.

RADIOLOGY

The radiographs of stress fractures of the femoral neck can be very difficult to interpret, particularly in the early—and important—stages without a good knowledge of the condition; only too often odd little appearances in elderly bones are dismissed too readily as being caused by age alone. The radiologist must be able to assess the radiological progress and diagnosis of stress fractures; Figures v.25 and v.26 show the radiographs of a woman of 81 who had pain in both hips for some while which had been worse over the last few months. The left knee was also painful. Examination showed slight limitation of movement with pain in the right hip but no pain in the left hip. There was slight flexion deformity in both hips but the knees moved freely. The original radiograph (Fig. v.25) shows a distraction stress fracture which was by no means united and which inevitably would continue to displace. This fact was not recognised

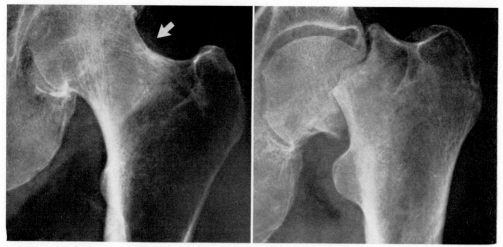

FIG. V.21   FIG. V.22

Figures v.21 and v.22 shows the radiographs of a woman, aged 76, who had had a long-standing osteoarthritis of the right hip which had caused her to take a great deal of weight on the left leg. Three weeks before seeking advice she had had considerable difficulty in standing with the weight on the left leg. Since then, she had either rested in bed or in a chair. The first radiograph taken six weeks before her symptoms began in the left hip showed the osteoarthritis in the right hip and the beginning of a stress fracture in the superior surface of the neck of the left femur (Fig. v.21). When she was seen again three weeks after the symptoms had started in the left hip, the fracture had become complete with considerable displacement which necessitated a replacement prosthesis (Fig. v.22).

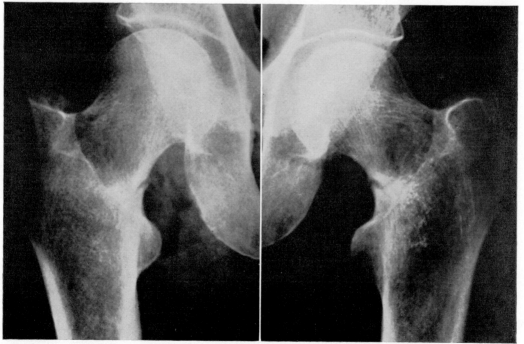

FIG. V.23   FIG. V.24

A woman of 68 years had pain in both hips. The radiographs show compression stress fractures. The patient was at rest in bed for three weeks until the diagnosis was established. She was then allowed up and made a satisfactory recovery without further treatment.

and the patient was allowed to walk. Four months later there was a definite further slip of the fracture which, fortunately, then became impacted. There is also evidence of a compression stress fracture starting at the level of the top of the lesser trochanter (Fig. v.26). This patient should have been treated by operation on the radiological prognosis because it is a distraction stress fracture.

It is of vital importance to get the best possible radiograph to help confirm the diagnosis. The radiographs shown in Figures v.27 and v.28 show the minutest crack in the superior cortex of the base of the femoral neck. This patient also had a severe osteoarthritis of the knee which, because of the stiffness or deformity therein, may predispose the femoral neck, or other parts of the leg such as the tibia, to fracture.

It is unusual to get a compression stress fracture of the femoral neck in an old person about which there would be no qualms on allowing the patient to walk; so it is not unwise to fix all such fractures in the elderly.

It is very rare for this fracture—of either type—not to be seen on the initial radiograph. This is different from most other stress fractures. Sometimes the displacement when first seen can be quite remarkable; particularly so when the patient is still able to walk as was the patient of whom the radiographs are shown in Figure v.29. She was 71 and had stumbled six weeks previously but had had pain in the left hip for only two or three weeks; when the radiographs were taken she had severe displacement of the fracture. The fact that there was no pain after the stumble indicates that this patient did not have a traumatic fracture. Figure v.30 is the radiograph of a woman who had pain in her right hip before she had fallen and sustained a Colles' fracture. Later increasing limp and pain made the patient seek advice for the hip.

Osteoarthritis known to exist may confuse the diagnosis which can perhaps only be made radiologically. Figure v.31 is of a woman of 61 who was diagnosed as osteoarthritic but in whom there was a stress fracture of the femoral neck. Again, Paget's disease near the hip can obscure the pain of a stress fracture nearby or even produce increased symptoms from a stress fracture-like lesion in the affected bone (Fig. v.32).

DIAGNOSIS

The diagnosis must be made on the history and examination and only confirmed by radiography, because, in the early stages, the stress fracture may be only just visible or not visible at all in routine radiographs. This is less likely to occur in the elderly but is most important in the young because of the outcome which can be crippling for life, particularly in that a chosen career may have to be abandoned because of the disability. Obviously the stress fracture that has become complete will have all the signs and symptoms of a fractured neck of femur. In the early stages there may be only the slight ache on weight-bearing and perhaps some pain on forced movement of the hip in some directions. The pain may be referred to the thigh or even to the knee. It is possible, in the more advanced stress fracture, to elicit deep tenderness around the femoral neck. The general examination is usually normal.

In the elderly the diagnosis must, as in the younger patient, rest on the symptoms and signs; fortunately it is rare not to get radiological confirmation of the stress fracture at an early stage and usually by the time the patient first presents. Against this, however, is the number of other conditions that beset the elderly, such as degenerative joint disease, rheumatoid arthritis, osteoporosis and suchlike that can confuse both the clinical and radiological picture. Even rest pain at night can occur to confuse the

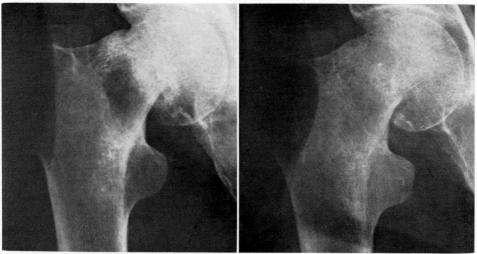

FIG. v.25   FIG. v.26

A woman of 81 had sustained a fracture of the left femur 30 years previously. Recently she had pain in both hips radiating down the thighs and into the left knee. The right hip had pain on attempting all movements other than flexion, of which it had a good range. The left hip had a free range of movement. The radiograph showed that she had a complete stress fracture of the right femoral neck which, at that time, was thought to be united (Fig. v.25). However, two months later there was no doubt that the position had altered and that union was still unsound (Fig. v.26). This explains why the movements of the hip were still very painful on the first visit, and emphasises the importance of the clinical findings.

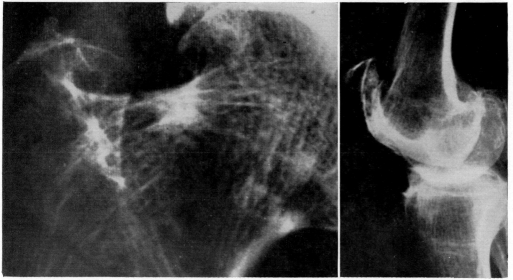

FIG. v.27   FIG. v.28

A woman of 88 developed pain in the right hip. She was greatly incapacitated by severe osteo-arthritis, particularly of the right knee, which somewhat detracted from the clinical appreciation of the painful lesion in the hip. However, the first radiograph of the hip was well positioned and care-fully exposed and showed without any doubt the beginning of a stress fracture in the superior cortex of the neck near its base (Fig. v.27). The radiograph of the knee confirmed the arthritis (Fig. v.28). This patient was treated by internal fixation and was able to return to the old people's home, whence she had been admitted.

I

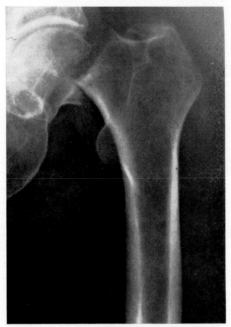

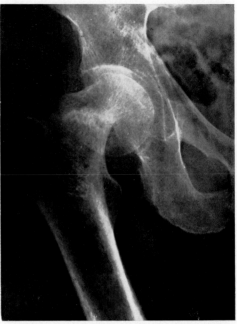

FIG. v.29

FIG. v.30

A woman of 71 had pain in her left hip for some three weeks. She gave a history of having stumbled three weeks before the hip started to be painful. When first seen she had a completely displaced fracture of the femur, on which she was still walking. At operation, when a replacement prosthesis was inserted, the ground-up bony tissue was white and soft and was sent for histology because it resembled neoplastic tissue. This patient exemplifies the difficulty of always being certain that trauma is in fact the cause of a fractured neck of femur. In her case the history was sufficiently clear to consider that the stumble did not in fact cause the fracture for she had three weeks with no pain in her hip before it began to ache.

A woman of 75 fell and sustained a Colles' fracture. Later she said she had had pain in her right hip before her fall. When the Colles' fracture had been treated, and some five weeks later, a radiograph was taken of the hip because she was beginning to limp badly. The stress fracture of the neck of the femur was quite old radiologically, and sections of the bone removed at operation for a replacement prosthesis showed some callus formation. She had a very severe osteoarthritis of the right knee with deformity.

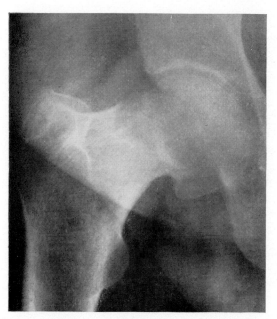

FIG. V.31

A woman of 61 had had pain in the right hip which had started insidiously, with no history of injury. The diagnosis clinically was osteoarthritis of the hip. The radiographs, however, showed a progressive distraction stress fracture of the femoral neck, which without treatment would continue inexorably to displace.

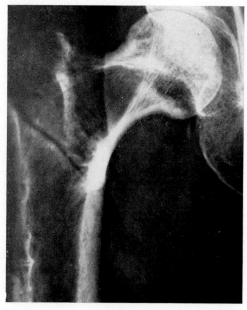

FIG. V.32

A woman of 76 with known Paget's disease was thought to have suffered a stress fracture of the right hip although there had been a history of some injury three weeks before the first radiograph was taken. She had been able to walk on the leg after the injury. After a further three weeks the radiograph above showed extension of the 'stress' fracture. There are also multiple 'stress' fractures lower down the shaft and it may well have been that one of these small fractures was increased by the injury.

The treatment for this fracture in Paget's disease is internal fixation if possible but the whole of the shaft of the femur should be examined radiologically lest a further fracture be found below the level of a radiograph positioned to show the hip.

problem. Spinal pain is often referred to the groin and may be present at the same time that a stress fracture is developing. All this emphasises yet again that, in order to be accurate in diagnosis, a full general examination is always necessary and a diagnosis must be made before resorting to radiology.

In many old people the stress fracture is diagnosed too late; too late because the weakened bone has, either with the ordinary activities of daily living or because of some slight twist or stumble, broken completely. In some patients great displacement can occur slowly and walking is continued, though with pain (Fig. v.29). In others the displacement is abrupt and the patient may fall to the ground. Thereafter the symptoms are, naturally, those of the ordinary fractured neck of femur.

In the same way that certain conditions predispose to stress fractures of the tibia in the elderly, notably osteoporosis, whether idiopathic or secondary to a definite cause such as rheumatoid arthritis treated with steroids, so is the hip liable to the same conditions. In addition the pelvis has often had high dosages of radiotherapy for malignant disease in the pelvis, and it is also a common site in which to find metastatic bone deposits. The latter problem is exemplified in Figures v.33 and v.34, in which are shown the radiographs of a woman of 52 who had had an adenocarcinoma of the ovary removed and followed by radiotherapy. The compression stress fracture might not be associated with either event, since it is seen at this age; but it is likely that radiotherapy had weakened the bone and rendered it more liable to a stress fracture.

Steroid treatment of rheumatoid arthritis or any other systemic condition produces bone that is extremely alike to that of the old person in the way in which it reacts to the everyday stresses of ordinary living; when a stress fracture occurs it follows the pattern in the elderly, particularly in the femoral neck as is shown in Figures v.35 and v.36. This patient also serves as a reminder that stress fractures are often bilateral but not necessarily at the same time.

TREATMENT

It is wise to accept that treatment is urgent in all patients with stress fractures of the femoral neck and that even those with compression stress fractures, whether young or old patients, must be considered for internal fixation unless there are good grounds for conservative treatment only. Figures v.35 and v.36 show what can happen to a fractured hip that is not diagnosed and treated soon enough. The best treatment in the old patient is, without doubt, to excise the hip and replace it with a prosthesis that can be cemented into place. Often the patient is osteoporotic and walking on the broken hip may cause non-union, as indeed can occur even in a younger age group. Because decubitus is very bad for patients with osteoporosis no matter how trivial, they must continue to be ambulant, and a replacement prosthesis is the quickest and safest way to achieve early walking after operation. Further, the liability of a trifin nail or other devices of a similar nature to fail is much higher than the usual failure rate for ordinary fractures. The trifin nail fixation in an osteoporotic neck of femur, particularly if the fracture is subcapital, is not indicated even with a traumatic fracture; the basal stress fractures may also be very difficult to treat by this method although the chance of success with the lower fracture is much better than with one high in the neck near the femoral head.

Figures v.33 and v.34 show that the radiological diagnosis may be difficult. The first radiograph indeed showed the earliest stage of a compression stress fracture across

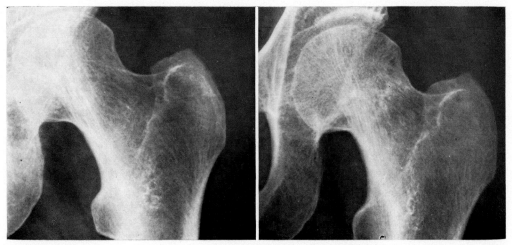

FIG. v.33   FIG. v.34

A woman of 52 complained of pain in the left hip. The year previously she had had an adeno-carcinoma of the ovary removed and had been put on to cyclophosphatase and had had deep x-ray therapy. When she first complained of pain she was fully investigated for secondaries and none were found. The radiograph of the left hip was thought to show no abnormality. Two months later the left hip was again radiographed because of the continuing pain and now the progress of the stress fracture can be seen very clearly. This is a compression stress fracture high in the neck which was probably caused in part by the irradiation osteoporosis. It was treated by a replacement prosthesis and no evidence of metastases were found in the specimen.

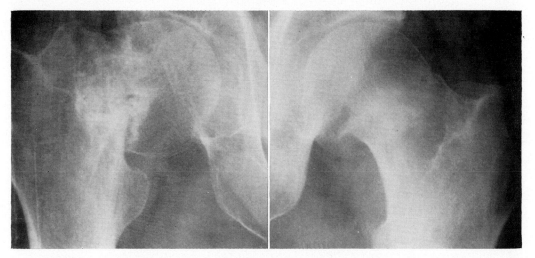

FIG. v.35   FIG. v.36

A man of 48 who had severe rheumatoid arthritis treated by steroids developed an increasingly severe pain in the right hip. The patient took to walking with a stick, and when first seen six weeks later the right hip had a badly displaced transverse stress fracture. It was not considered possible at that time that it could be reduced and the fracture was allowed to unite in the displaced position (Fig. v.35). The patient was warned that the opposite hip could suffer the same condition, and one year later he returned with a similar but not quite so severe pain in the left hip with no history of injury. He had come to hospital at once. The radiographs showed an early transverse stress fracture and this was successfully treated by internal fixation. It is interesting that, although the patient attended quickly, there is displacement in the first radiograph shown in Figure v.36 and this would undoubtedly have progressed to the same displacement as the opposite hip.

the neck, but this was not appreciated and it was thought there was no abnormality, apart from the osteoporosis. Two months later there is an obvious stress fracture developing across the subcapital area of the neck. This was considered to be a post-radiation type of stress fracture of the femoral neck and was treated by a replacement prosthesis. Even if pinned this fracture will invariably proceed to disintegration of the femoral head.

Stress Fractures of the Femoral Head

Stress fractures of the neck of the femur can be subcapital, mid-cervical or basal, as has been seen. The highest fractures are comparable to those traumatic fractures which involve the head itself. If a compression stress fracture occurs in the head of the femur it is possible that this blocks the blood supply to a part or the whole of the femoral head. It has been demonstrated that stress fractures occur more frequently in patients with rheumatoid arthritis, particularly when treated with steroids, than in the normal person. Thus it might be expected that if a compression stress fracture was to occur in the lower part of the femoral head it would occur more frequently in patients with rheumatoid arthritis treated with steroids. 'Steroid' arthropathy is known to occur in which the collapse of the femoral head has been attributed to some effect of the steroid. This, of course, is true in that the steroid has reduced the strength of the bone by causing osteoporosis and so the likelihood of a stress fracture has been increased. Figures v.37 and v.38 show the radiographs of the femoral head of a patient of 73 who had severe rheumatoid arthritis which had been treated by steroids. She had many aches and pains, but the pain in the right hip had started abruptly a few months after the radiograph shown in Figure v.37 was taken, and then became very severe. Further radiographs were taken, it now being eight months after the previous radiograph, which showed that the upper part of the femoral head had collapsed (Fig. v.38). It is possible, when comparing the two, to see that there is a line of internal callus in Figure v.38 at the bottom of the portion of the head that has collapsed, and this line can also be seen in the previous radiograph (Fig. v.37). The onset of symptoms probably coincided with the beginning of the collapse. The pre-existing compression stress fracture within the head has damaged the blood supply and caused a partial avascular necrosis.

Figures v.39 and v.40 show two radiographs of a woman of 60 who developed increasing pain in the left hip. She had chronic rheumatoid arthritis and had been treated by gold five years previously and by steroids for three years. In the first radiograph (Fig. v.39) the head of the femur has a distinct and easily seen fracture line running across it, with a slight amount of displacement. To substantiate this the alteration in the lines of force as shown by the trabeculae in the femoral neck have altered and do not have the normal splay and direction to fit those in the acetabulum. At the upper and outer part of the stress fracture, and just below it, there is callus which can be seen quite clearly. There has, as yet, been no collapse, nor is there any very great change in the density of the femoral head. One year later the final outcome is seen in the radiograph in Figure v.40. The head has been destroyed from the line of the stress fracture shown in the first radiograph to leave only the medial and lower part of the femoral head.

The destruction that occurs sometimes in an osteoarthritic hip may also develop in

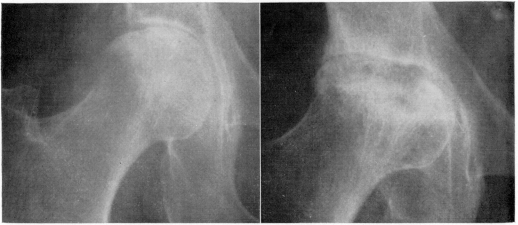

FIG. v.37   FIG. v.38

A woman of 73 had been treated with steroids for severe rheumatoid arthritis. Quite suddenly her right hip started to ache. A radiograph had been taken some eight months previously (Fig. v.37) and had been passed as normal. The radiograph taken when she complained of the increase of pain showed a progressive collapse of the femoral head (Fig. v.38). There is a line of internal callus below the level of the collapse, and careful examination of the earlier radiograph (Fig. v.37) shows that there is some internal callus to be seen on the thicker band of trabeculae running upwards through the centre of the head. A compression stress fracture has caused avascularity of the upper and central part of the head, which has collapsed.

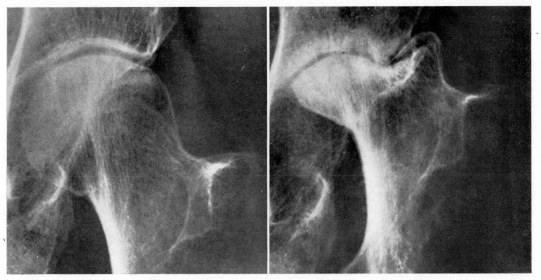

FIG. v.39   FIG. v.40

A woman of 60 developed pain in her left hip. She had had chronic rheumatoid arthritis for many years and had been treated by gold injections and then steroids. With no injury she developed a painful hip. In the first radiograph, shown in Figure v.39, there can be seen a stress fracture of the upper and outer aspects of the head of the femur, which curves across until it disappears above the centre of the head. There is also slight displacement. Figure v.40, taken one year later, shows that the head of the femur has been lost from that point on the upper, outer, aspect of the head where the fracture line can be seen in the previous radiograph. There is some internal callus just below the upper and outer end of the fracture line seen in the radiograph in Figure v.39, and also the lines of the trabeculae have altered and do not fit—as they should—those in the acetabulum; there is also a suggestion that they have angled at the level of the stress fracture.

the same way. Figures v.41 to v.43 show the radiographs of a woman of 76 who had osteoarthritis of her left hip. The original radiograph in Figure v.41 shows a compression stress fracture running transversely across the base of the femoral head. Eight months later, as is shown in Figure v.42, this fracture line is less obvious but the outline of the area which will ultimately collapse is already clearly visible. Figure v.43 shows the final outcome when the patient was admitted for a total hip replacement.

The stress fracture has been shown to compress at times and in the osteoporotic patient a thin break across the head of the femur, slightly compressed, could very easily be sufficient to block the blood supply either by causing venostasis or by actual involvement of the small arteries passing up through the cancellous bone. It is of interest to note that stress fractures in the neck of the femur occur in the elderly in much the same way as do stress fractures of the pubis. The latter also are seen in children in whom, instead of a stress fracture of the femoral neck, there occurs a slipped upper femoral epiphysis; but in the younger age group Perthes' disease is seen. This is discussed in Chapter Ten.

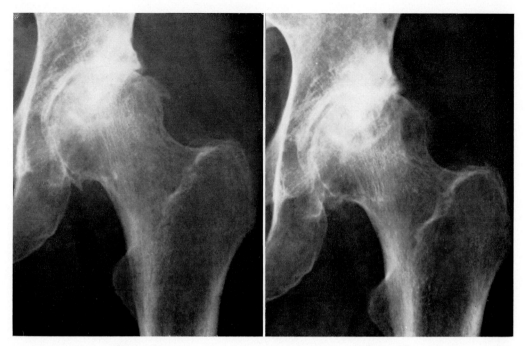

FIG. v.41   FIG. v.42

A woman of 76 had severe osteoarthritis of
her left hip (Fig. v.41). Some seven months
later the radiograph showed increasing dis-
organisation (Fig. v.42). The two radiographs,
when compared, show that there has been a
compression stress fracture running almost
horizontally across the centre of the head of
the femur and that this has, in part, disappeared in the next radiograph shown in
Figure v.42, but there is already the outline of
the avascular upper part of the femoral head.
When the patient was admitted for a total
hip replacement the destruction was complete
(Fig. v.43).

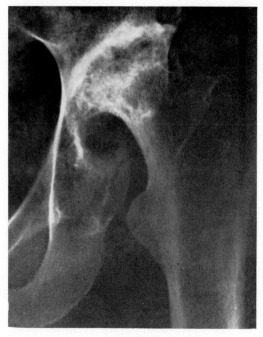

FIG. v.43

CHAPTER SIX

STRESS FRACTURES OF THE PATELLA

One important aspect of stress fractures in the patella in the adolescent or young adult is the emphasis it puts on the stresses that are applied to that bone. True stress fractures of the patella are seen either passing transversely across the lower half of the body or running distally down the lateral aspect. Stress fractures of the patella have not been seen over the age of 30 years. In the child the stress that occurs around the patella may cause a fracture of the lower pole but more commonly causes an avulsion of the attachment of the patella ligament with or without a flake of bone. A bipartite fragment may be partially avulsed to cause slight separation of the fragment and considerable disability. It is possible that the bipartite fragment is, in some cases, the late result of avulsion of a part of the patella. A more detailed description of avulsions in general and of the patella in particular is given in Chapter Ten but some examples are given in this chapter to show how stress fractures merge into 'osteochondritis' or avulsions of the lower pole of the patella.

The patella takes no weight; the cause of its stress fracture is purely muscular, the pull of the quadriceps muscle being resisted by the patella ligament.

Sometimes, particularly in the stress fracture that runs transversely across the body of the patella, operation is needed to prevent—or correct—displacement and in all patients immediate treatment is necessary. An example of a stress fracture running across the body of the patella is shown in Figures VI.1 to VI.3, which are the radiographs of an athletic young doctor. The original stress fracture can be seen in Figure VI.1 and the separation that occurred within a very short time is shown in Figure VI.2. At operation, fortunately, it was possible to return the fragments into excellent position in which they united as is shown in Figure VI.3.

The symptoms and signs that occur in the child with a stress lesion of the lower pole of the patella are the same as those that occur in the condition known as 'osteochondritis', or the 'Larsen-Johansson syndrome'. The bipartite patella, when causing symptoms due to partial separation, is best treated by excision of the fragment.

SYMPTOMS AND SIGNS

The patient is invariably active whether a young adult or a child. No stress fracture has been seen in the patella in a person not undertaking some form of special activity.

The history is of pain of rapid onset after or during a period of activity or sport. This may have been preceded by a dull ache for some days during activity. At first the pain is not very severe and rarely is there swelling unless the stress fracture involved the joint, when there may have been a haemarthrosis; but because the patella occupies a very special position in regard to the stability of the knee, and as it is one of the few sites of a stress fracture that actually involves a joint directly, symptoms are often severe enough to necessitate early advice. The child or adolescent, on the other hand, can have a long history of a painful knee, particularly if the symptoms come from a

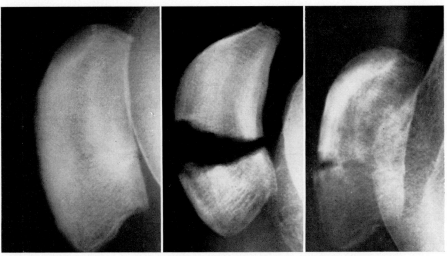

FIG. VI.1   FIG. VI.2   FIG. VI.3

A doctor of 28, a fast runner and a centre forward at hockey, was playing tennis when he felt pain in the knee. He attended hospital the same day and the radiograph confirmed a stress fracture running across the patella (Fig. VI.1). He was admitted to hospital but before operation the pain got worse because the patella had become separated at the fracture site (Fig. VI.2). Repair, using absorbable material, was satisfactory (Fig. VI.3) and the patient made an uninterrupted recovery. These radiographs show the danger of not treating the patella stress fracture immediately.

FIG. VI.4 An athletic man of 25 who was in training had to enter hospital to have his tonsils out. After this he had two weeks holiday and then returned to training. After one week he had an aching discomfort in the right kneecap but with no swelling. He then played football and for the first hour of the game the knee continued to ache. He jumped to head a ball and, on landing, something clicked in the lower part of his knee and he found he could not stand well but he managed to continue the game with further pain in the knee. The next day the knee was swollen and he was found to have a transverse stress fracture of the lower pole of the patella. He still had full movements at that time except for being unable to lock his knee into full extension with the usual snap. After three weeks in a plaster cylinder the fracture had united and a further month later he could run three miles without discomfort.

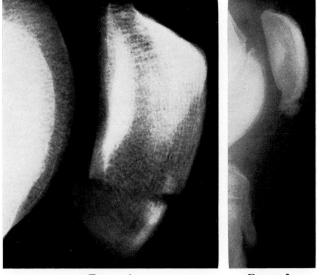

FIG. VI.4   FIG. VI.5

FIG. VI.5 A schoolboy of 13 was doing sport when his knee began to hurt while running and jumping. The diagnosis of an 'Osgood-Schlatter' syndrome was made but the radiograph showed that he had a stress fracture of the lower pole of the patella. This healed very satisfactorily. Six weeks later the boy did develop an osteochondritis of the tibial tubercle of the same knee.

bipartite patella. It is at this stage that careful examination will find tenderness localised to that part of the patella affected.

Figure vi.4 shows a very similar stress fracture to that shown in Figures vi.1 to vi.3 but it is a little lower down in the patella. This patient was a man of 25, an athlete, who had his training interrupted to go into hospital for removal of his tonsils. After he took a short holiday, he returned to training. After a few days he felt an aching in the right kneecap but there was no swelling. He then played football and for the first part of the game the knee continued to ache. After jumping to head a ball he felt on landing that something had clicked in the lower part of his knee and he could not stand up very well, but he managed to continue the game with more pain. The next day the knee was swollen and he sought advice. He was diagnosed as having a stress fracture of the lower pole of his patella. Apart from being unable to lock the knee into full extension with the usual snap he had full movements. It is interesting that the lower pole of the patella had actually separated and displaced slightly but was still firmly against the remainder of the patella; it united without further trouble. Fortunately the fracture did not involve the joint surface.

The same history is present in the younger patient but may be longer. Figure vi.5 shows the patella of a schoolboy of 13. His knee began to hurt while doing sport. He was diagnosed as having osteochondritis of the tibial tubercle but the radiograph showed that he had developed a stress fracture of the lower pole of the patella. A few weeks later it had healed satisfactorily but the tibial tubercle then developed pain and tenderness. In the younger patient the two conditions of a stress fracture at the lower pole of the patella and a stress lesion of the tibial tubercle are closely associated; this is fully discussed in Chapter Ten.

In the stress fracture of the lateral side of the patella the symptoms are much the same. Figure vi.6 is the radiograph of the patella of a student of 23 who gradually developed pain in his left knee, particularly while doing long-distance running in his recreation. Before the pain he had done rather more than usual cross-country running. He was quite adamant that there had been no injury, no locking and no giving way of his knee. A short while before attending for treatment he had run for a bus and the pain became worse and he felt a click in the knee which became swollen and painful. The first radiograph (Fig. vi.6) shows that he had a stress fracture of the lateral lip of his patella. A radiograph three months later (Fig. vi.7) showed further, if slight, displacement. At operation to excise the fragment there was only fibrous union but the histological examination of the fracture surface showed callus (Fig. vi.8).

The examination of a patient with a stress fracture of the patella is made easy by the fact that the whole of the patella on its subcutaneous surface and most of the deep surface can be palpated directly. There should be no difficulty in localising the tenderness to the exact part which has sustained the fracture, the knee being otherwise entirely normal apart from a haemarthrosis if it is present.

RADIOLOGY

Careful radiology is needed in all patients to ensure that a small lesion is not missed. Figures vi.6 and vi.7 show that the fracture was quite obvious in the tangential views but it could hardly be seen in the ordinary anteroposterior and lateral projection.

The patella must have at least three radiographic views, the two normal anteroposterior and lateral projections as well as a tangential view. Figures vi.9 and vi.10

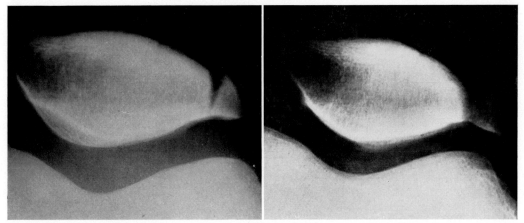

FIG. VI.6   FIG. VI.7

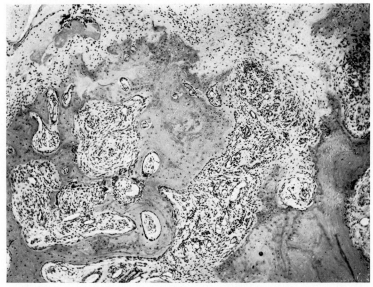

FIG. VI.8

A male student of 23 gradually developed pain in the left knee. He was a long-distance runner and in the spring had done a great deal of cross-country running; in December of the same year symptoms started. He was adamant that there was no history of injury, no locking and no giving way but a short while before coming to hospital he had had more pain on running for a bus. There was a click and the knee became swollen and painful. He was tender on the lateral aspect of the left patella only and the radiograph (Fig. VI.6) showed a stress fracture of the lateral margin of the patella. Three months later he still had symptoms (Fig. VI.7); he was admitted for operation at which fibrous union was found between the patella and its smaller lateral fragment which was excised. Some four months after leaving hospital he was back in full training with full movements and no symptoms. The two radiographs show that the displacement had increased slightly while the patient was having conservative treatment. The histology of the surface of the small fragment (Fig. VI.8) shows new bone formation and ossification in provisional callus.

show the tangential and lateral radiographs of the bipartite patella of a boy of 16. The tangential radiograph showed a definite difference between the two patellae from which it was deduced that the bipartite fragment had been pulled away from the remainder of the patella. Provided the radiological examination is complete and carefully done it is usual for a stress fracture or similar lesion of the patella to be readily confirmed. Figures VI.11 to VI.14 show that the bipartite patella giving symptoms can show a difference to the opposite patella which, though bipartite, is symptomless.

DIAGNOSIS

In the younger child the diagnosis is difficult at times since it may be thought that the child has chondromalacia of the patella, and if the symptoms persist for some while, as they may with the lesions around the lower pole or with the bipartite type of patella, it may be difficult to distinguish between the two. However, the very careful examination will locate the tenderness exactly and it will then be found to correspond with the lesion seen in the radiographs. The boy of 16 whose radiographs are shown in Figures VI.9 and VI.10, and who was already working as a bank clerk, played a lot of sport. Despite conservative measures over a considerable period of time, he continued to complain. The original diagnosis was thought to be chondromalacia at that time but the localisation of his symptoms to the fragment of the patella which does seem to have moved out of position, as is seen particularly in the lateral radiograph, led to exploration and excision of the fragment with complete resolution of symptoms. There is no doubt that a very careful and prolonged examination of the patella must be undertaken and familiarity with the technique of feeling the patella on all its surfaces is essential to making an accurate diagnosis. The length of symptoms in the adolescent must not preclude that there has been a form of stress fracture.

In the very young child, such as the one whose radiographs are shown in Figures VI.15 to VI.19, the history of the pain occurring with exercise or after exercise must make one suspicious of a stress fracture. In her case the lower poles of the patellae were affected and the left side was the worst. A small flake of bone could be seen to have been separated from the lower pole of one patella, to be followed by the same appearance in the other. In fact the flake is ossification in the partially avulsed patellar tendon origin, because the right patella showed no flake at first, although the symptoms and signs were present. Another example in a young child is shown in the radiographs in Figures VI.20 to VI.22, which show the patella of a girl of 11 who noticed that her left knee started to hurt after doing a long jump but that it did not hurt during the jump. It became painful and swollen and she was tender around the whole of the patella. A careful history elicited the fact that it was not the actual jumping that hurt but that it came on after the jumping and that three weeks previously she had had a similar but milder episode. Figure VI.20 shows the normal right knee and Figure VI.21 the left knee at the time of first being seen. After six weeks the fragment had united firmly by bone, as is shown in Figure VI.21, and she was free of symptoms. The patients in the two last examples had similar symptoms and signs; one pulled off a fragment of the bone with the patellar tendon and the other the tendon from the bone.

The differential diagnoses include another derangement of the knee, osteochondritis of the tibial tubercle, rupture of the tendon of the rectus femoris and an infrapatellar bursitis. All these can be distinguished early on the history and examination. An exception is chondromalacia of the patella or of one or both femoral condyles, especially

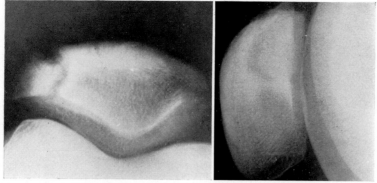

FIG. VI.9   FIG. VI.10

A lad of 16 who was working in a bank played a lot of sport and developed pain in the right knee in which he had a bipartite patella. Despite intensive conservative treatment his symptoms continued. Figure VI.9 shows that the bipartite fragment is no longer in a normal relationship to the remainder of the patella, and this is confirmed by the lateral radiograph shown in Figure VI.10. At operation the fragment was excised with complete resolution of all symptoms and he returned to full sport.

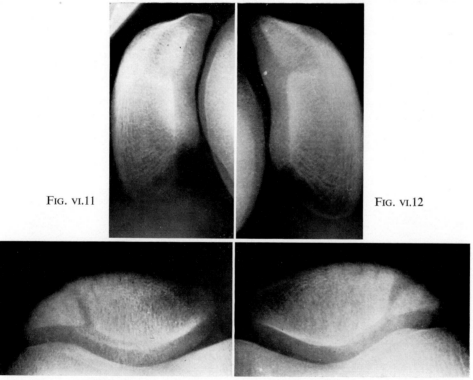

FIG. VI.11   FIG. VI.12

FIG. VI.13   FIG. VI.14

A boy of 16 with bilateral bipartite patellae developed a painful right knee after strenuous athletics three days before being seen. Clinically he had a stress fracture of the right patella—based more on the history than on the examination, since he was quite certain that he had no pain during his athletics but that it came on gradually afterwards. He had tenderness over the centre of the patella with fluid in the joint but no other findings were noted. The radiographs showed a definite difference between the right (Figs. VI.12 and VI.14) and left (Figs. VI.11 and VI.13) patellae in the tangential and lateral views. Excision of such a fragment offers the best hope of early return to full function.

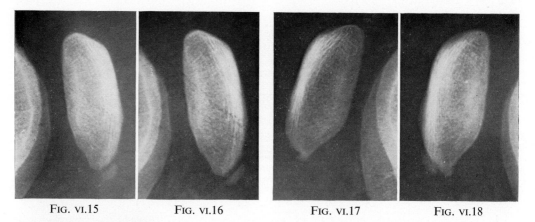

FIG. VI.15   FIG. VI.16   FIG. VI.17   FIG. VI.18

FIG. VI.19

FIG. VI.15 to FIG. VI.19

A young girl complained of swelling of the left knee which she had had for one month with pain which she located in the lower part of the patella. She also had some pain in the right knee but less so than in the left. Activity made it worse. The lower poles of the patella were tender but the left was the worst. Otherwise she had a full free range of movement. The only other finding was a mild physiological genu valgum. The first radiographs show a flake from the lower pole of the left patella (Fig. VI.15) but the right patella seemed normal (Fig. VI.17). Two months later the flake at the lower pole of the left patella has increased in density (Fig. VI.16) while a similar appearance is present in the right (Fig. VI.18). The girl was treated by rest from all activities that hurt and she was better in six weeks. Two years later the patellae were normal (Fig. VI.19). This series of radiographs shows that the 'flake' at the lower pole can be caused by ossification in the haematoma caused by the patellar tendon being pulled off its origin by stress with exactly the same symptoms and the same cause as a stress fracture.

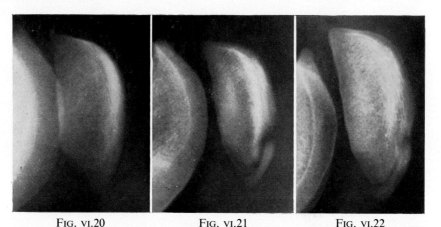

FIG. VI.20   FIG. VI.21   FIG. VI.22

A girl of 11 noticed that her left knee started to hurt after doing the long jump and she was insistent that it did not hurt during the jump. It had become painful and swollen and she was very tender around her kneecap. She was able to walk afterwards but she said she had had a similar pain in the same knee three weeks previously and probably even before that. Figure VI.20 shows the normal right patella. In Figure VI.21, the first radiograph, it can be seen that the lower pole of the left patella has had the bony attachment—or anterior cortex—avulsed. She was treated in a plaster splint for six weeks, at the end of which time she was quite better (Fig. VI.22). There has been a stress fracture through the lower part of the patella where the patellar ligament is attached.

that over the fragment of an osteochondritis dissecans in its early stages, which can be very difficult to distinguish from a stress fracture. The pain from chondromalacia is very similar to that caused by a bipartite patella that has displaced, so similar in fact that it is probably the joint cartilage over the fragment that gives as much in the way of symptoms as does the syndesmosis.

TREATMENT

For the transverse stress fracture in the body or the lower pole of the patella immediate immobilisation is necessary, with the knee almost straight to relieve all strain on the patella. This is achieved most easily with a plaster cylinder from groin to ankle, and the patient may weight-bear in it because if the patella stress fracture has not separated, the quadriceps expansion will not have been torn and will control what pull there is from the quadriceps muscle. On the other hand, if separation has occurred, then it is necessary to operate and to reduce the fracture and fix it with some satisfactory method to prevent displacement. The patient shown in Figure vi.1 to vi.3 had the patella sutured together with thick catgut. The patient in Figure vi.4 was treated in a plaster cylinder for three weeks.

The younger child with the stress fracture or avulsion at the lower pole will usually respond adequately to desisting from activities that bring on the pain. If the child is too active and does not take the instruction to rest seriously then immobilisation is necessary if only to achieve this rest.

The bipartite patella is alleged not to give rise to symptoms but in fact when displaced, even very slightly, by stress it is necessary to excise it and this can be done through a small incision with little morbidity from the operation. The small fragment can be cut away from the rest of the patella with the knife but sometimes the apparently easily followed line of syndesmosis in the radiograph is very different to that which has to be followed by the scalpel. The attachment of the synovia and capsule is sewn back as best possible and the patient may get up and weight-bear without a plaster as soon as straight-leg raising can be achieved, which is within two or three days.

DISCUSSION

The patella, although not carrying weight, transmits a very strong force from the quadriceps muscle to the patella tendon; it has the two forms of stress fracture either in the lateral part or horizontally and because it is part of the knee joint early effusion is often seen. The exception to this is in the lowest part of the patella which is outside the joint. Thus often the child with the fragmentation of the lower pole of the patella has no effusion. Because the patient may attend quite quickly after the onset and because the examination if not done with the utmost care may reveal little wrong, radiographs may not be taken and the wrong treatment instituted with a disaster in that the fragment separates.

In the younger patient with a bipartite patella it may be pulled apart slightly. When this happens excision of the fragment cures the symptoms and returns the patient rapidly to full activities, and early operating is advocated.

That the lower pole of the patella obtains stress fractures in adolescents can be traced back to the young child in whom the lesion is often considered to be a fragmentation of the lower pole of the patella or osteochondritis. However, it is clear that the latter condition is in fact a stress avulsion of the attachment of the patella tendon to the patella and this is discussed further in Chapter Ten.

K

CHAPTER SEVEN

STRESS FRACTURES OF THE PELVIS

Stress fractures of the pelvis occur in the inferior ramus of the pubis in both adults and children (Figs. VII.1 to VII.3). Less often it is seen in the superior pubic ramus or in the body of the pubic bone near the hip, although only in adults. Bilateral stress fractures are common in children, in whom the pain may resemble that of hip disease. Adolescents do not get stress fractures of the pelvis; instead they have avulsions near the hip, especially in the iliac spines and in the ischial tuberosity, and the occurrence is associated with activity. The latter are dealt with in Chapter Ten.

The stress fracture in a child is very similar to that found in the older person but it is most interesting that these stress fractures have not been seen between the ages of about 11 to 60 years, when they start to occur again usually in women of whom some have associated osteoporosis or other disability such as rheumatoid arthritis.

Stress Fractures of the Inferior Pubic Ramus in Children

The importance of this condition is firstly that the symptoms and signs may closely resemble hip disease and secondly that it is common. The diagnosis of this fracture in a child does not eliminate a coexisting disease of the hip, therefore great care must be taken and the child kept under review until all symptoms have gone. An accurate history from child and parent, a careful examination, and a clear understanding of the clinical and radiological findings will give sufficient confidence in the diagnosis so that the child need not be admitted for observation of the hip.

SYMPTOMS AND SIGNS

The child, more often a boy than a girl and between 5 and 10 years old, is brought for advice with a history of some weeks or even months of pain in the groin, a limp, or even of only walking sufficiently badly to cause parental anxiety. The symptoms may have increased over the previous week or two, with tiredness of the child as a whole or in the leg in particular. The parent may have noticed a falling-off of activity and the child is said to be listless and always wanting to sit or rest. Sometimes there has been some incident, such as a childhood tumble, to which reference is made but which caused no true injury.

Both the inferior pubic rami are often affected although the complaint is on one side only. This is because the most painful side limits activity so that the side least affected does not hurt; however, there are occasions when a child complains of both sides. Therefore both rami may be tender.

For the examination the child must be calm and relaxed, warm but fully undressed. It is impossible to examine a child who is cold or crying, anxious or apprehensive. With the child supine there will, rarely, be noticed some wasting; but gentle palpation

138

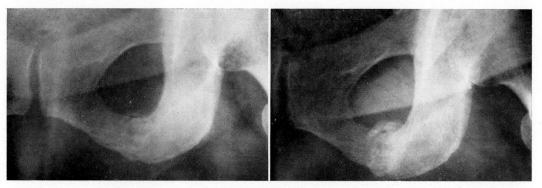

FIG. VII.1   FIG. VII.2

A woman of 66 had noticed a little pain in the region of the left hip for a week or two before she spent three hours at a church service. After this the pain in the left hip became very severe with all movements of the leg and hip being painful. She was hardly able to get home. The radiograph (Fig. VII.1) taken a few days later shows a stress fracture of the inferior pubic ramus. One month later the radiograph (Fig. VII.2) shows that the fracture is consolidating.

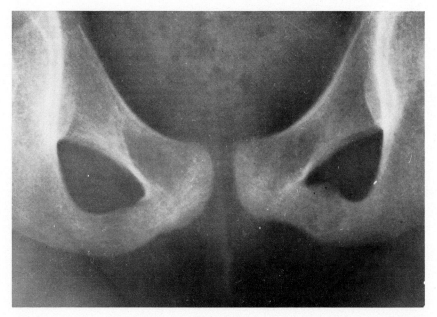

FIG. VII.3

A doctor's daughter aged 8 had had pain on and off for several months in the left hip region but it was always worse after exercise. She located the pain quite accurately into the left groin and she was very tender over the inferior pubic ramus. The radiographs show the stress fracture of the left inferior pubic ramus.

will find a point of considerable tenderness near the centre of the inferior pubic ramus on one or both sides. The tenderness is at the origin of the adductor muscles, which, when stretched, cause pain and discomfort in the stress fracture which can be confused with pain in the hip. The thickening of the inferior pubic ramus cannot be felt although it is seen radiologically to be considerably enlarged; this enlargement is apparent in Figures VII.4 to VII.6, the radiographs of a boy aged $8\frac{1}{2}$ with bilateral stress fractures, and the progress of the lesions is shown.

Wasting of the affected limb can be easily recognised and may cause difficulty in finding the correct cause. Figure VII.7 shows the radiograph of a boy of 5 who had a limp and quite marked wasting of the thigh and calf. No other lesion was found besides the stress fracture nor did any other condition appear during follow-up. Bilateral stress fractures may cause wasting in both legs, but which may then not be recognisable.

RADIOLOGY

The development of the callus in a stress fracture of the inferior pubic ramus can be quite remarkable, with considerable heaping up and an almost bubbly formation in the new bone, as can be seen in Figures VII.8 and VII.9 in which it will be noted that in the earliest radiograph, when the boy was 6, the ischiopubic cartilage had already united by bone. There is a slight enlargement on the opposite side which may well have been another fracture that did not develop because the lesion on the right had slowed up activity. The second radiograph (Fig. VII.9) shows healing, and the angular fracture line can be seen running upwards and medially, first through the inferior surface of the ramus then at right angles upwards and outwards and finally medially to the upper surface.

Radiographs suggest that this type of stress fracture is one of compression rather than distraction. It might at first glance seem that the normal stresses in the ischio-pubic rami and in the superior pubic ramus would be that of distraction—or tension —but the hip, the lower end of the femur and the pubis together make a triangle which must have compression between the pubis and the hip if the latter is not to abduct. Particularly will this be so in the normal action of walking or running.

In Figures VII.10 to VII.12 the gonadal shield is shown which is a hazard in the radio-logical diagnosis because it may be wrongly placed and so screen the lesion. The radiographer must use the proper shield correctly placed so that the pubic bones are visible in both boys and girls.

DIAGNOSIS

The important condition from which a stress fracture must be differentiated is hip disease. The age at which the fractures occur, being from 5 to 10, includes Perthes' disease, tuberculosis, acute or chronic infective arthritis and osteomyelitis. The tuber-culous hip, still prevalent in some parts of the world, may start with similar symptoms but the muscle spasm of a stress fracture is soon relieved with simple rest without traction, and examination done properly will exclude the hip as being at fault. The low fever which is present occasionally from haematoma absorption lasts only a few days; it is usually irregular and never very high.

Slipped upper femoral epiphyses do not come into the differential diagnosis because of the age, and stress fracture of the neck of the femur is never seen before the upper femoral epiphysis is closed. Certain other stress fractures in the area should not cause

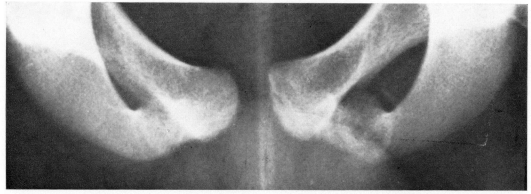

Fig. VII.4

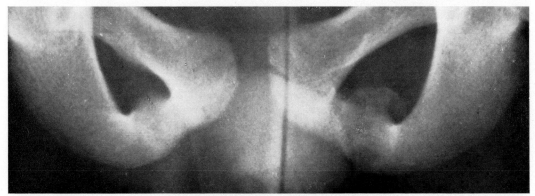

Fig. VII.5

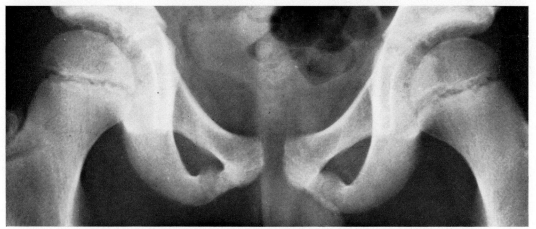

Fig. VII.6

A boy of 8½ years had had pain in his left hip for some while but the exact time was unknown. The hip was found to be painful in full abduction, full flexion and full lateral rotation and was tender at the left inferior pubic ramus only. The radiograph showed a stress fracture with much callus on the left with perhaps a similar condition on the right (Fig. VII.4). The next radiograph (Fig. VII. 5), three months later, shows consolidation of the callus on the left and an increase in the amount on the right. The final radiograph (Fig. VII.6), at six months, shows the smoothing down of both rami but the fracture lines can still be seen.

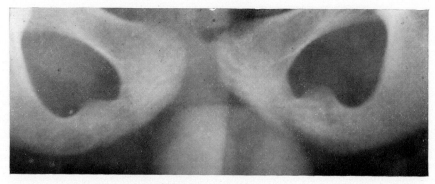

FIG. VII.7

A boy of 5½ was referred with a limp in the left hip. Examination showed that he had slight wasting of both calf and thigh with tenderness over the inferior pubic ramus. The diagnosis of a stress fracture was made and confirmed radiologically. There is the suspicion of another stress fracture beginning on the other side but it gave rise to no symptoms.

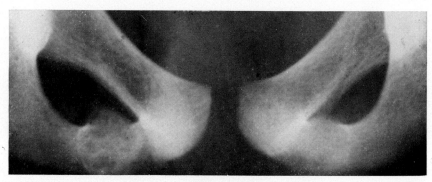

FIG. VII.8

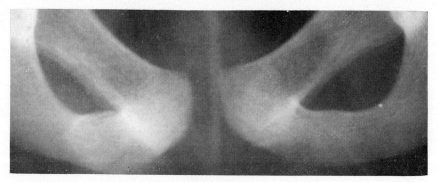

FIG. VII.9

A boy of 6 was referred with a peculiar gait. He walked with knock knees and rotated the right leg inward more than the left. He was found to have limitation of lateral rotation of the right hip. The initial radiograph (Fig. VII.8) shows callus around the inferior pubic ramus. Two months later the symptoms and signs had settled completely, but the line of the stress fracture can now be seen (Fig. VII.9).

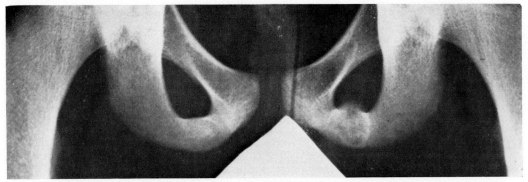

FIG. VII.10

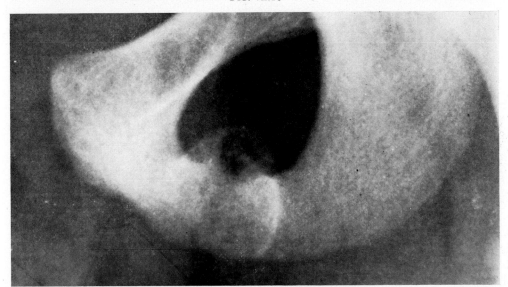

FIG. VII.11

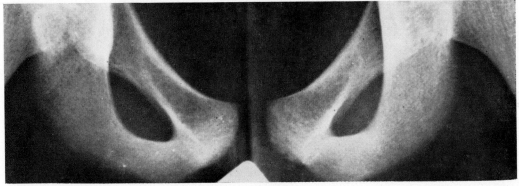

FIG. VII.12

A boy of 8 was referred to hospital because of an undescended right testicle, and pain in the left hip for one month which had caused him to limp. The testis was in the superficial inguinal canal and the radiograph showed a stress fracture of the left inferior pubic ramus (Fig. VII.10). The right ramus was normal. Three months later, in Figure VII.11, the callus is much enlarged, but eight months later, in Figure VII.12, it can be seen that the bone has returned to normal.

confusion since they occur at a different age, such as those at the anterior iliac spines, lesser trochanter, acetabular lip or ischial tuberosity.

TREATMENT

No treatment is necessary other than to reassure parents and child and to confine activity to within the limits of pain. That this regime does ease the child of pain must be checked carefully, to ensure that there is no other condition present. For the more severe pain a few days rest in bed will help, with gradual return to activity afterwards. The normal life of a child, including school, should be continued but without taking part in games, sport or walking to a sufficient extent to cause pain.

With rest all stress fractures of the pubis in children heal rapidly within one to two months, at the end of which time the child is back at full activity which needs no further curtailment. As with other stress fractures of childhood no systemic abnormality is to be blamed for the condition; rather it occurs in the more active child than in the less athletic.

Stress Fractures of the Pubis in the Elderly

In the adult, stress fractures occur over the age of 60 and usually after some unaccustomed activity as was the case of the patient shown in Figures VII.1 and VII.2. Perhaps this fracture occurs in women because the shape of the female pelvis is different from that of a male or because of the greater tendency to osteoporosis.

The fractures may occur in the inferior or superior pubic rami, on the same or the contralateral side, and, in the osteoporotic patient, in all four rami.

SYMPTOMS AND SIGNS

The pain comes on gradually and increases with activity. No patient will have had an accident bad enough to fracture the pelvis, but many patients will inculpate a knock or jolt as the cause of the increased symptoms. The pain is felt in the groin but often it is said to be in the hip. It may go down the side of the thigh, even to the knee. It is always worse during or after walking, which, at times, is prevented by the severity of the pain. Untoward movement may hurt; resting in bed does not always relieve the patient completely, as is usual with other forms of stress fracture, because it is difficult for the adult to lie in one position without causing some strain on the pelvis. Particularly is this the case in those patients in whom both the superior rami and inferior rami are involved on the same side.

Walking can be very painful in some patients with more than one rami fractured, so that a stick or a walking frame is used.

There will always be tenderness at the fracture sites, which can be located with considerable accuracy in either rami. Distraction of the fractures by pressing on both the anterior superior iliac spines with the patient supine will cause discomfort, but this test must be done with care as it can cause very severe pain if done roughly. Because of spasm, the muscles may also be tender locally. There will be free movement of the hip when it is carefully examined but any pull on muscles or ligaments that strain the fracture site will cause pain.

Examination of the hips and lumbar spine will, at this age, often show arthritis or other degenerative conditions, which must not detract from the careful assessment of the sites in the limbs at which stress fractures occur.

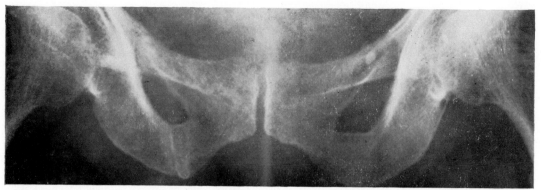

Fig. vii.13

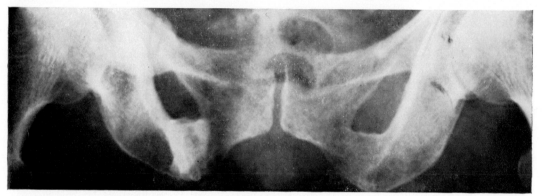

Fig. vii.14

A woman of 65 developed pain in the right groin which went down to the knee. Previously she had had some backache. She had a severe limp and was very tender over the right pubic region. The clinical diagnosis of a stress fracture was confirmed radiologically. There is a fracture at the origin of the superior pubic ramus from the body of the pubis, as well as in the inferior pubic ramus of the same side. Further investigations as an out-patient revealed no abnormality other than a mild degree of idiopathic osteoporosis. She made a good recovery.

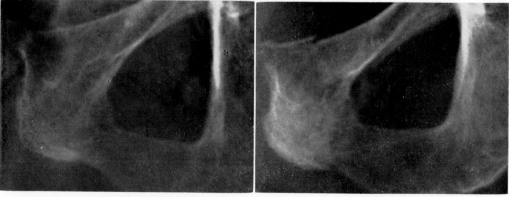

Fig. vii.15   Fig. vii.16

A woman of 69 complained of pain in the left buttock and groin after a long car journey. She also had rheumatoid arthritis but had not been treated with steroids. She remained resting for a week after the journey but was then admitted to hospital for further investigation because the first radiograph (Fig. vii.15) was passed as normal. Three weeks later the fracture was clearly visible. It is at the origin of the rami from the body of the pubis (Fig. vii.16). The patient made an uninterrupted recovery with simple curtailment of those activities which caused pain.

RADIOLOGY

The fracture will be difficult to see early on but it is clearly visible in four to six weeks, at the time the patient usually presents. If the fracture is seen in the radiographs at the first visit a careful history will have recorded that there has been a slight ache for several weeks; this is often lost because of an acute episode engendered by some trivial incident to which the patient attributes the pain, and the slight ache that preceded it is forgotten.

The radiographs of the pelvis must be very carefully positioned and exposed. Other conditions in the older person, such as arthritis of the spine, may prevent the patient from lying supine without the very careful placing of cushions or pillows.

The radiographs of a woman of 65 are shown in Figures VII.13 and VII.14. There has been a stress fracture of both superior and inferior pubic rami; it is usual to find that the superior ramus has its stress fracture either at the junction of the body with the ramus or at the other end, close to the symphysis pubis. This is shown in Figures VII.15 and VII.16.

DIAGNOSIS

The history of low back pain or arthritis of the hip may confuse, because with both the pain is worse with activity and rest pain may occur in the same way that pain from a stress fracture is often felt after activity. However, these conditions are usually simple to discard by the clinical examination. A stress fracture of the femoral neck must be excluded. Gynaecological complaints that might cause similar pain are rarely seen in these patients; but painful herniae are to be excluded.

Neoplasms can cause weakening of the bone, with pain which is, at first, identical to a stress fracture; this is because the weakened bone does, in fact, allow a stress fracture to occur. Any unusual form of fracture, which is thought to be caused by stress, must be suspect.

TREATMENT

Bed rest should be avoided in the elderly and particularly in the osteoporotic patient. Limited activity must be encouraged. If walking is painful, sticks or a walking frame should be given. It is much better for the elderly patient with a stress fracture of the pubic rami to walk in moderate comfort using a frame than to be chair-bound with no pain. Suitable analgesics are of great help, particularly in the early morning to allow dressing and toilet in comfort, and at night to ensure sound sleep. The pain, which is often occasioned by getting out of a chair, can be much improved by either using a high chair, raising the chair on a plinth or using an ejector seat. This allows the patient to rest at will without the fear of pain. A full explanation of the cause of the pain is most helpful since most patients will accept some pain if they do not have to suffer anxiety about it as well. Local injections and pelvic supports have little beneficial effect.

In the otherwise healthy patient recovery is quick and it does not take long for the stress fracture to unite, but the more osteoporotic the patient the more difficulty there will be in the assessment of how soon the patient will be active. Figure VII.17 shows the radiograph of an aged nun in whom the number of stress fractures was so great that the pain enforced complete rest in bed from which she never rose again. In contrast Figure VII.18 shows a single stress fracture of the superior ramus which united with simple restriction of activity.

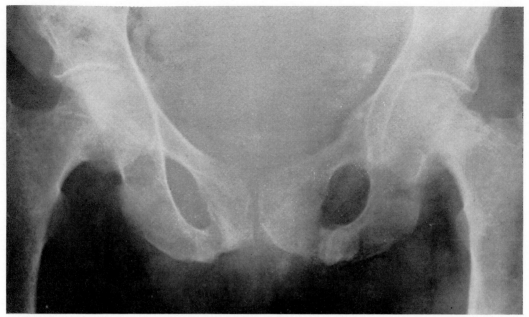

FIG. VII.17

A nun aged 84 had been bedridden for no very good reason except general aches and pains. She complained of increasing pain in the left hip and groin, and the radiograph shows stress fractures of the left femoral neck, at the junction of the superior ramus of the left pubis with the ilium, in the inferior pubic ramus and there is also another stress fracture starting in the right femoral neck. Later, further stress fractures were found in the right pubic rami. The patient declined treatment and remained bedridden until she died.

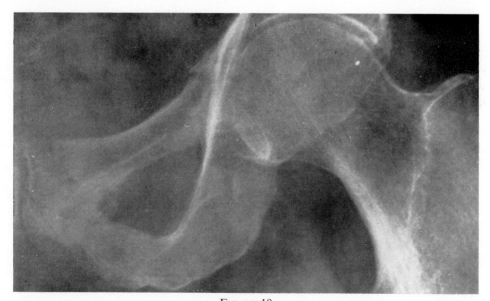

FIG. VII.18

A woman of 60 had diabetes and Parkinsonism and looked older than her age. She had pain in the groin, which she had first noticed when pushing a sofa some distance along the floor. The radiograph shows that there is a stress fracture at the junction of the superior ramus with the body of the pubis. This healed satisfactorily with rest from activities and furniture moving.

CHAPTER EIGHT

STRESS FRACTURES IN THE FOOT

The bones of the foot that have been seen to be affected by stress fractures are the calcaneus, the navicular bone, the metatarsal bones and the sesamoids of the great toe. The calcaneus gets a compression stress fracture as does the first metatarsal bone at its proximal end, while the three middle metatarsal bones get in particular oblique stress fractures, which at the beginning are comparable to those seen in the fibula but also they have compression stress fractures at the neck or actually in the metatarsal head. The fifth metatarsal bone often sustains a transverse or distraction stress fracture near its base with displacement. The navicular bone has an atypical type of stress fracture which, although quite distinctive when it occurs, is probably exceedingly rare. A stress fracture in a sesamoid bone is believed to be a true entity but again they are not often seen, perhaps because of failure in diagnosis, this being difficult, as is its radiological confirmation.

The complexity of the structure of the foot and the different muscular forces that are applied to each part in the normal mechanism of walking or running explain the variety of stress fractures seen and, in diagnosis, very careful attention to the history and the examination will usually lead to the correct clinical diagnosis.

Stress Fractures of the Calcaneus

Stress fractures of the calcaneus in adults occur at any age and often account for the painful heel that eludes diagnosis because of the vagueness of the symptoms and the failure of the radiological changes to be found early. Perhaps the calcaneus has the longest latent period in developing radiological confirmation of a stress fracture and three months is not too long to wait. A similar stress fracture occurs in the apophysis at the calcaneal tuberosity in children.

SYMPTOMS AND SIGNS

The patient has almost invariably had a period of increased exercise or some unusual (but not abnormal) activity to induce the pain; it can start fairly abruptly, with swelling of the hind foot and general disability. Figures VIII.1 to VIII.4 show such a fracture. In the radiograph taken three weeks after the patient had gone for a long walk on hard roads (Fig. VIII.1) the line of internal callus is seen. The second radiograph (Fig. VIII.2) some two weeks later shows the development of the fracture across the trabeculae. The tangential views in Figures VIII.3 and VIII.4 show the density of the callus, with a slight amount of external callus on the medial border which is more readily appreciated when compared with the normal, left, side in Figure VIII.3.

By the time of attending for advice, the patient has probably lost the swelling around the ankle but will have great tenderness under the ball of the heel and also on each side

148

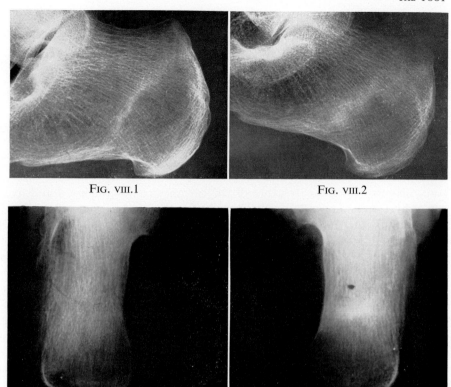

FIG. VIII.1

FIG. VIII.2

FIG. VIII.3

FIG. VIII.4

A woman of 47 went for a long walk along a road and developed pain in the ankle. It was moderately severe and there was swelling of the ankle. The symptoms continued for three weeks until she was first seen. The haze of internal callus can be seen in the radiograph in Figure VIII.1 running at a right angle to the trabeculae near the junction of the tuberosity with the body. After a further two weeks the callus is seen more clearly in the radiograph (Fig. VIII.2). The tangential views in Figures VIII.3 and VIII.4 show the callus formation in the right calcaneus, with some external callus on the medial border. The density of the internal callus is well seen when the affected calcaneus (Fig. VIII.4) is compared to the normal (Fig. VIII.3).

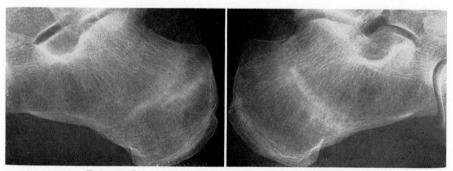

FIG. VIII.5

FIG. VIII.6

Radiographs of a woman of 71 who had done a lot of extra walking and over several months developed pain in both heels. They show that she had developed bilateral stress fractures. That on the right conforms to the pattern of a double stress fracture quite close to the tuberosity; on the left there has actually been compression, particularly at the superior part. Some callus lies externally at the fracture line. The patient responded well to simple treatment, including thick sorbo heel pads.

of the body of the calcaneus at its junction with the tuberosity. It is here that the fracture occurs. The tuberosity itself, in the adult, is not tender. Movements of the foot and ankle will be full and free passively but the patient may be unable to stand on the heel with the forefoot off the ground or unable to stand on the toes without considerable exacerbation of the pain. Careful examination will exclude all other lesions that are to be found in the adult, particularly in the calcaneal tendon, which, if suffering from an incipient rupture, may mimic the pain distribution. The pain of plantar fasciitis may also cause difficulty but it is more localised than that of a stress fracture to one point in the ball of the heel.

RADIOLOGY

The confirmation of a stress fracture of the calcaneus is long delayed and may not show even in an elderly and osteoporotic patient for two or three months. The general outline of the fracture is an area of internal callus which can often be double. This haze of new bone usually stretches all the way from the junction of the body of the calcaneus to the tuberosity in its upper part, downwards and forwards towards the inferior surface. In older patients, when they are perhaps osteoporotic, the compression may actually show, as is the case in Figures VIII.5 and VIII.6 which are the radiographs of a woman of 71 who had done a lot of extra walking and who had developed, over several months, pains in both heels. She was thoroughly investigated because of the osteoporotic appearance of her bones. She had sustained bilateral stress fractures of the calcaneus, worst on the left, and she responded well to simple heel pads of soft rubber in the shoes. The progress and healing of such a fracture is shown in Figures VIII.7 to VIII.9.

DIAGNOSIS

The diagnosis of a stress fracture of the calcaneus is based on the symptoms and signs. The increased activity preceding a painful heel or ankle with pain lasting many months is the usual finding. Swelling of the hindfoot is not usual when the patient presents, unless attendance is exceptionally soon after the symptoms have started. The most important finding is pain produced by the effort of standing on tiptoe, when the forces engendered compress the tuberosity of the calcaneus against its body. Next in importance, and to which great attention must be paid, is the location of the pain in the heel, and, although the ball of the heel will be very tender, there will be extreme tenderness at the sides of the body of the calcaneus over the line of the stress fracture. This tenderness is higher than that found in plantar fasciitis. No radiological confirmation need be expected before several months have passed, often about three, and if treatment has been effective during that time only very slight changes will be seen in the radiographs.

The important differential diagnosis in a stress fracture of the calcaneus is the over-enthusiastic diagnosis of a plantar fasciitis or calcaneal spur and its treatment by hydro-cortisone injections which, of course, have no effect. The tenderness of plantar fasciitis can always be localised, almost to a point source in much the same way that the lateral epicondylitis can also have a point of source of tenderness. The stress fracture of the calcaneus is very much more diffuse but, if examination of the patient is cursory and the whole of the heel not carefully palpated, local tenderness will be elicited only under the ball of the heel and a wrong diagnosis made. There is always tenderness on both

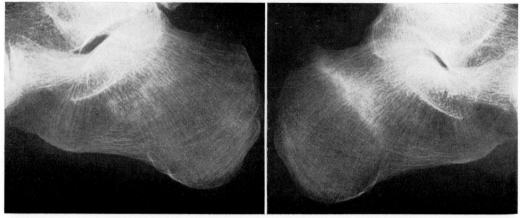

FIG. VIII.7   FIG. VIII.8

FIGS. VIII.7 to VIII.9   A woman of 67 had had three weeks pain in her left heel. She also had had a similar pain in the right heel five weeks previously but it was less severe and had only lasted a week or two. The pain in the left heel got steadily worse each day, particularly after walking. She noticed that walking flat-footed caused less pain than walking properly. Swelling was always present around the heel at night but was better in the morning. Examination showed that both calcanei were extremely tender to pressure on their lateral aspects and in the centre of the tuberosity. Forced plantar flexion caused pain in the left heel. The patient was a diabetic but was otherwise healthy. The radiograph on the right, or painless, heel at this time showed that there had been a stress fracture that was already disappearing (Fig. VIII.7). The left calcaneus has a double stress fracture (Fig. VIII.8) which is more obvious in Figure VIII.9 six weeks later. This patient had the very frequent double fracture in the body of the left calcaneus. Bilateral calcaneal stress fractures are also common but, as shown by this patient, the less affected side may pass unnoticed.

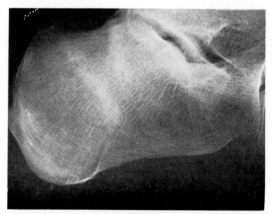
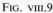
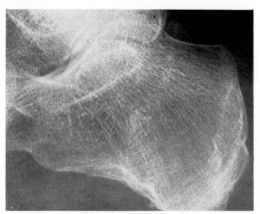

FIG. VIII.9   FIG. VIII.10

FIG. VIII.10   A woman of 80 fell and injured her right hip. She had pain in the heel which she said she had had before her fall, and a casual examination of the radiograph suggested a stress fracture in the right calcaneus. Attention to detail shows that this is the superimposed shadow of a calcified artery.

sides of the heel and usually at the back of the heel over the tuberosity. Gout must be excluded and the swelling of the heel which may be present may cause some suggestion of a local inflammatory condition. The rupturing calcaneal tendon must be carefully excluded because of the description of the pain and its referral to the back of the heel, but the localisation of the tenderness will be sufficient to differentiate the two conditions. The tibial tunnel syndrome and other types of tenosynovitis may cause pain which, being occasioned by activity, may cause confusion. Other stress fractures of the lower end of the tibia or fibula or in the foot must also be excluded. The ache of the 'dropped arch' is easily excluded by inspection and palpation of the foot as a whole.

The radiological appearances are very easy to understand once it is appreciated that they are slow to occur. Occasionally local calcification in an artery can mislead in the older patient. The calcified posterior tibial artery may mimic the compression stress fracture in a remarkable way. Such a one is shown in Figure VIII.10 in a woman of 80. The pain in the heel of which she complained after she had fallen was diagnosed as a stress fracture after it had been seen in the lateral radiograph but it is in fact the superimposed shadow of the calcified artery.

TREATMENT

Treatment by means of a soft rubber pad in the heel of the shoe is usually sufficient, sometimes helped by strapping the foot and ankle. Probably the pad, by raising the heel, is more efficacious by virtue of reducing the compressing force of the calf muscles and long plantar ligament on the calcaneal tuberosity than by the softness of the rubber.

DISCUSSION

The cause of a compression stress fracture of the calcaneus is in no doubt and has been dealt with in Chapter One and Figures I.26 to I.29. The fracture is not caused by banging the heel on the ground in running or walking but through compression of the body of the calcaneus by its tuberosity, the compression of force being the pull of the calf muscles inserted into the tuberosity resisted by the long plantar ligament. This is why the line of the fracture is invariably curved across the line of the compression, which is more vertical in the superior part and more horizontal in the lower part.

Stress Fractures of the Calcaneus in Children

Stress fractures of the calcaneus in children occur in the apophysis. The fracture does not take the same form as in the adult, perhaps because the cartilage between the calcaneus and the apophysis absorbs some of the stress that passes inwards from the apophysis. This leaves the apophysis in much the same position in regard to stress as is the patella with the knee bent. The so-called osteochondritis of the heel is in many cases a stress fracture of the apophysis, and Figures VIII.11 to VIII.18 show a bilateral example in a boy of 10.

This fracture in the child gives rise to a history of some weeks' pain in the heel, worse with exercise as would be expected, and after the child walks or runs there is a complaint of pain.

Examination shows that only the point of the heel is tender. The radiographs will show fragmentation in one or the other plane of the apophysis. If the radiograph is taken at the height of the symptoms it may well suggest that there is a fragmentation

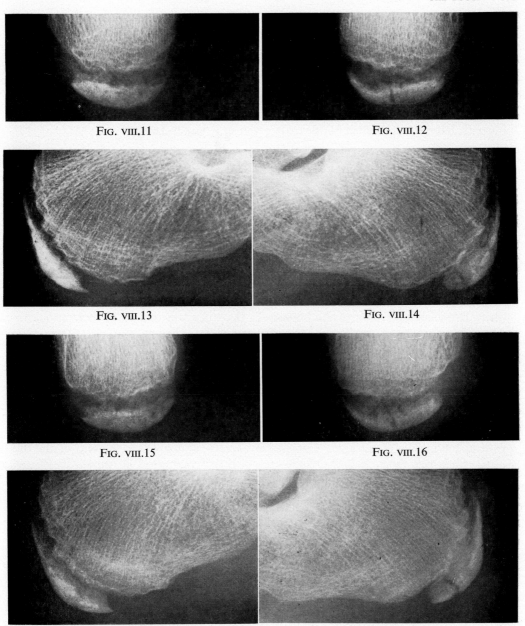

FIG. VIII.11

FIG. VIII.12

FIG. VIII.13

FIG. VIII.14

FIG. VIII.15

FIG. VIII.16

FIG. VIII.17

FIG. VIII.18

A boy of 10 had painful heels for two months. Examination showed that there was tenderness over the ball of the heels but nothing else was found. He was treated with heel pads and strapping and after some weeks he was quite better. The original tangential radiographs (Figs. VIII.11 and VIII.12) show the apophyses in which the fracture is shown more clearly on the left than on the right. Two weeks later, in Figures VIII.13 and VIII.14 the fracture on the left is seen well in the lateral radiograph; in the right there is a suggestion of a crack in the apophysis which is denser than the left. The tangential radiographs taken at the same time (Figs. VIII.15 and VIII.16) show the fracture in the left apophysis. Three months later the apophysis on the right has healed but the left still shows the lower stress fracture although the upper fracture has healed (Figs. VIII.17 and VIII.18). The very thick periosteal covering prevents callus from showing on the surface of the apophysis.

L

but the illustrations in Figures VIII.11 to VIII.18 show that the fracture lines can be clear-cut.

The treatment is simple; the child will be perfectly comfortable if the shoes have a firm thick sorbo pad put in the heel. Excess activity is curtailed for some two months; there will then be freedom from symptoms. Careful attention to this condition will prevent at least some, if not all, cases being diagnosed as osteochondritis of the calcaneal apophysis.

Further discussion of osteochondritis is given in Chapter Ten.

Stress Fractures of the Navicular Bone

It is rare to see a stress fracture of the navicular bone. Although the radiological appearance is of a linear fracture running distally from the talonavicular joint, through the centre of the navicular bone, it is in fact a compression stress fracture.

Despite the fact that no big muscles are inserted into the navicular bone, the muscular pull on the forefoot has to be resisted by the medial arch of the foot and, when standing on tiptoe, the forces passing through the medial border of the foot are greater than the actual weight of the body because, added to gravity, there is the tension in the muscles —which causes compression of the bones—so that they will remain in their appointed position. The force from the head of the talus passes into the concavity of the navicular bone which is then pushed apart.

The counterpart of this stress fracture in childhood is a form of juvenile avascular necrosis caused by the blood supply of the bone being damaged by the internal callus of a compression stress fracture.

SYMPTOMS AND SIGNS

Pain in the middle of the foot, worse after exercise and towards the end of the day is usual. Such was the case in the right foot of the woman aged 60 shown in Figures VIII.19 and VIII.20, a keen golfer. For a woman of her age the examination showed no abnormalities of note, provided that the moderate degree of hallux valgus is accepted as not an abnormality and is not considered to be a predisposing factor. This particular patient had to be treated in a below-knee walking plaster cast as it is difficult to withdraw the stress on the navicular bone by asking the patient not to do those things which cause the pain. Once this fracture has occurred simple standing can make the foot ache towards the end of the day. Therefore complete rest had to be ensured by a tight-fitting below-knee cast.

The history of pain in the foot is so common in middle age that at first the connection between this and a stress fracture will be missed unless emphasis is always made on asking when the pain occurs. Once the connection with activity has been discovered it is likely that the metatarsal bones will be considered as perhaps having a stress fracture, but examination will show that there is none of the usual tenderness. The fact that the pain is on the medial side of the foot will make the examination of the first metatarsal bone important, but again the tenderness will be found to be more proximal. Ligament strain and flat foot will be seriously considered unless the point of greatest tenderness is found lying around the dorsum, the medial border and, to a less extent, the inferior border of the talonavicular joint. As is usual in the foot, very careful examination is needed to exclude the various strains that may have occurred to the ligaments round the ankle joint and in the foot itself.

Standing may not cause pain, at least in the early part of the day; the patient may well have a flat-footed stance on the affected side and care must be taken to be certain the opposite foot is not also affected. Standing on tiptoe may be painful.

RADIOLOGY

The navicular bone in the adult when it develops a stress fracture has only been seen to have the simple crack passing in a longitudinal direction from the centre of the articular surface of the talonavicular joint in the sagittal plane. This is shown in Figures VIII.19 and VIII.20 and also in Figures VIII.21 and VIII.22. The fracture in the navicular bones are identical. In the radiograph in Figure VIII.22, taken some six weeks after the first, the fracture can be seen to be healing.

TREATMENT

The pain of a stress fracture usually comes on during or, at a variable time, after exercise. However, in the case of the navicular bone it is almost impossible to prevent pain occurring with any form of activity so that even simple standing, which puts considerable stress through this bone, causes aching. Therefore it is necessary to relieve the foot of much of the weight-bearing stresses, and the patient may need a well-fitting below-knee walking plaster cast to prevent the pain. Strapping is insufficient treatment for this fracture unless the patient can withdraw enough activity from the daily routine so that the foot is rested.

Provided the plaster cast is properly applied and fits well then, although weight still passes through the navicular bone, it is a passive weight with far less muscular activity with considerably reduced stresses on the foot. As has been seen in Figures VIII.21 and VIII.22, healing is moderately rapid and had occurred after six weeks treatment.

DISCUSSION

This rare but interesting lesion in the navicular bone must be remembered in the adult in the same way as Köhler's disease is remembered in treating the painful foot in the child. Very early careful history-taking and diagnosis will reveal the suspicion of the condition.

March Fractures

A march fracture is a stress fracture of a metatarsal bone. The most common fractures are those that occur in the second or third metatarsal shafts. The symptoms of pain and aching in the forefoot are quickly relieved by rest and adhesive elastic strapping in practically all patients with march fractures, though not without exception.

It is difficult to assess how many march fractures do not follow the usual pattern. This is because the usual stress fracture of a metatarsal shaft is so readily diagnosed and so easily treated by the patient's practitioner—or gets better with slight restriction of activity without the benefit of medical advice—that it is usually the more severe fractures that are referred to hospitals for advice. The emphasis in regard to march fractures must, therefore, be placed on the more unusual metatarsal stress fractures which do

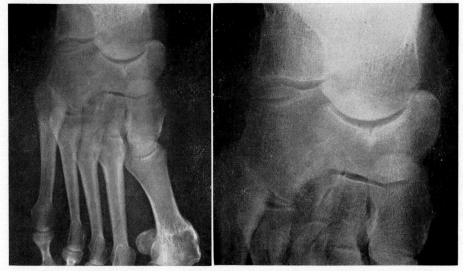

FIG. VIII.19   FIG. VIII.20

A woman of 60 complained of pain in the medial side of the right foot which she had noticed was much worse on playing golf. The pain had come on very gradually and she had had no injury. The original radiograph in Figure VIII.19 shows a stress fracture of the navicular bone which runs distally in the sagittal plane from the centre of the proximal articular surface. It does not go through the whole of the body of the navicular bone, and in the enlarged view in Figure VIII.20 the dense bone around the anterior end of the fracture line is well shown. It took several months for this patient to regain freedom from symptoms even with treatment in a below-knee walking plaster.

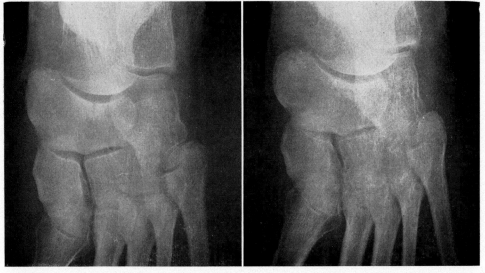

FIG. VIII.21   FIG. VIII.22

A woman of 66 gave a very accurate history when she was seen in December, saying that she had fallen downstairs in February and was much bruised, but although her left foot was painful it was quite well in two weeks. The patient then moved to a new district in June and the foot became painful and swollen, particularly on the anteromedial aspect. It was put into a below-knee walking plaster a few weeks after the onset of symptoms and this allowed the fracture to heal moderately quickly, probably because it had been caught earlier than the patient in the previous radiographs in Figures VIII.19 and VIII.20. Six weeks later the radiograph shows healing (Fig. VIII.22).

not conform to the established pattern and which may not respond in the usual way to simple treatment. Sometimes the disability—both temporary and permanent—caused by a march fracture can be considerable.

Multiple march fractures are the most common variant. Sometimes the outer three metatarsal bones will sustain stress fractures either together or in sequence. Bilateral march fractures occur but are rare because even if both feet sustain a march fracture at the same time the slight limitation on activity occasioned by that which becomes more advanced will allow healing to take place in the least affected side before the development of overt symptoms and signs in the other foot. In multiple march fractures it is usual to find that the third metatarsal bone is more often involved than not, followed closely by the fourth metatarsal bone.

Any part of a metatarsal bone may have a stress fracture; but the neck is less often affected than is the centre of the shaft. The base is rarely affected except in the first and fifth metatarsal bones in which a different mechanism is involved, and if the stress fracture actually occurs in the metatarsal head in a child it causes the condition known as a Freiberg's infraction.

The predisposition of a foot to a march fracture after it has been operated upon for some other condition, such as a bunion, is not accepted as proven.

One of the interesting features about the four lesser metatarsal bones is that when deformity occurs with a stress fracture there seems to be no consistent reason as to why the deformity should be medial or lateral in any particular patient.

Although the march fracture is most usually seen in the middle-aged adult the adolescent and young adult also get this stress fracture, usually with much sporting activity, including, of course, soldiers who go for long marches.

There is no doubt that unusual activity will produce the condition; it is the service recruit who will get a march fracture when he first starts long marches; it is the unaccustomed day out walking and shopping that will cause it in the middle-aged adult.

A march fracture has been called by more names than any other stress fracture—perhaps in more ways than one—but no point is seen in perpetuating the miscellany.

One of the problems with any metatarsal stress fracture is that ordinary standing is activity, and therefore for some patients pain, although more severe on walking or running, may also be considerable while standing at ease; thus weight-bearing has to be stopped to give complete relief. All age groups from 4 years old onwards are susceptible to march fractures. Sex has no obvious relationship to occurrence, and although the activity of the patient has considerable importance some patients get march fractures doing practically nothing.

The radiological confirmation of march fractures is not usually as long delayed as at some other sites and is usually present at two weeks.

The clinical and radiological findings of metatarsal stress fractures are described under separate headings for each bone; thereafter treatment is given for the group as a whole.

Stress Fractures of the Second Metatarsal Bone

The second metatarsal is the one most often affected by a march fracture. It has many variations in its presentation.

SYMPTOMS AND SIGNS

An ache or pain in the forefoot is the usual presenting feature, which may have been related to some special activity (classically a 'march') such as a day's outing, an extra long walk or a rather tiring game of golf. The pain gradually increases in intensity each day but it is possible for the patient to continue walking, sometimes limping, sometimes flat-footed—taking all the weight on the heel—sometimes hobbling on the inner or outer border of the foot. Running will be almost impossible because of the pain.

In a few patients the pain comes on abruptly. Close questioning may reveal a history that previously the forefoot had been aching slightly, but this is not always so. A small child may complain of a diffuse pain on the inner border of the foot, worse on walking. Such a patient is shown in Figure VIII.23: although only aged 4, he complained that his foot hurt if he went for long walks but it did not if he was on a short walk. The radiograph shows very clearly the stress fracture of the second metatarsal bone of the right foot which was already healing two weeks after symptoms began, when the child first presented. An older child, shown in Figure VIII.24, was sent for radiography by his doctor because, although he was thought to have 'strained' his foot recently, his doctor wondered if the symptoms were from a march fracture; the latter is shown very well in the radiograph in which it already appears to be healing well some three weeks after the onset of pain. The site of both the march fractures was the centre of the metatarsal shaft.

Inspection of the foot will show that swelling may or may not be present. Rarely is it obvious over the affected side. More often it will be general over the forefoot and, in some elderly people, the whole of the forefoot and even the ankle may swell.

Palpation will reveal tenderness localised to the second metatarsal shaft. It may be very difficult to be certain that it is the second and not the third metatarsal bone that is tender so careful examination with a gentle index finger is needed. Pressure under the forefoot may cause pain and manipulating the bone by holding its head gives rise to pain. Standing on tiptoe is painful. Swelling along the shaft of the bone is not felt even in the early case. Figure VIII.25 is the radiograph of a girl of 20 who had only had symptoms for ten days. The distal part of the second metatarsal shaft has a stress fracture slightly comminuted and displaced. No swelling could be felt clinically.

RADIOLOGY

The radiological appearances appear to bear no relation to the signs or symptoms but nevertheless they are extremely interesting. Sometimes it takes some weeks for the radiographs to show the fracture, and Figure VIII.26 is the radiograph of the second metatarsal bone with a stress fracture that had been present for three weeks. There is callus but the fracture line can hardly be seen. However, in the stress fracture shown in Figure VIII.27, which is the radiograph of a woman who had had symptoms for only ten days, the fracture line is clearly seen but there is no callus of note. Figure VIII.28 shows a different type of stress fracture that has a long fracture line running up the shaft. In this patient, as might be expected, pain even after one month was still causing sufficient trouble to necessitate a plaster cast.

The three last-mentioned figures (VIII.26 to V.III28) show how different the radiological appearances may be, from simple callus formation in Figure VIII.26 to the clear-cut oblique crack in Figure VIII.27 and the longitudinal fracture line in Figure VIII.28.

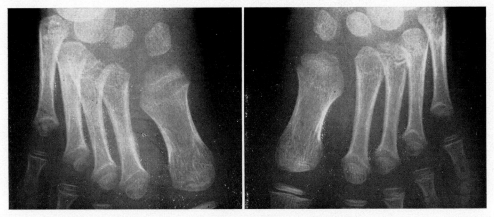

FIG. VIII.23

A boy of 4 complained of pain along the inner border of his right foot, which was worse on long walks. The radiograph confirmed that he had a stress fracture of the second right metatarsal shaft which was already healing. Symptoms lasted about two weeks.

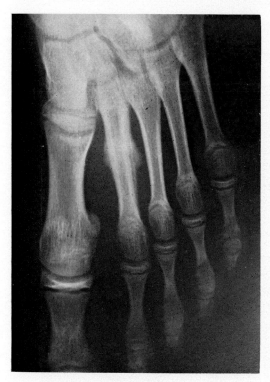

FIG. VIII.24

A boy of 12 was referred to hospital with a diagnosis of a march fracture. In the radiograph the subperiosteal callus and that outside the periosteum at the actual fracture site is shown.

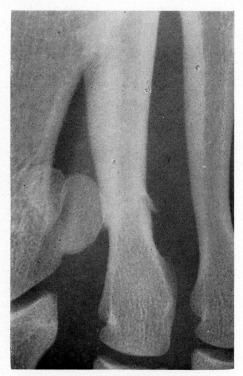

FIG. VIII.25

A girl of 20 had pain in her foot. There was no swelling clinically or radiologically but much tenderness. The stress fracture is not only complete but is comminuted with slight displacement.

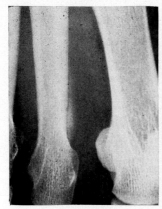
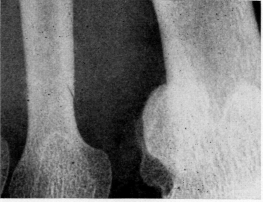
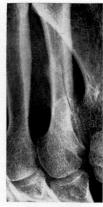

FIG. VIII.26   FIG. VIII.27   FIG. VIII.28

FIG. VIII.26   A woman of 32 had had sudden onset of pain three weeks before attending for advice. Despite this, when the radiograph was taken only a haze of new bone was to be seen on the medial aspect of the lower metatarsal shaft.

FIG. VIII.27   A woman of 46 spent some time on a ladder painting her house. The next day she felt some pain in her foot and when she attended for radiography some ten days later an oblique crack could be seen in the medial cortex of the lower part of the metatarsal shaft. However, careful inspection will show that the lateral border has a step in it so this fracture must be complete.

FIG. VIII.28   A woman of 48 had a history of pain in the foot for one month, and because it failed to improve with simple measures, she was put into a below-knee plaster cast. The oblique radiograph which is seen here shows that the fracture is longitudinal up the shaft. Perhaps because it never became a complete fracture it was still stressed with every step so that the pain continued to get worse.

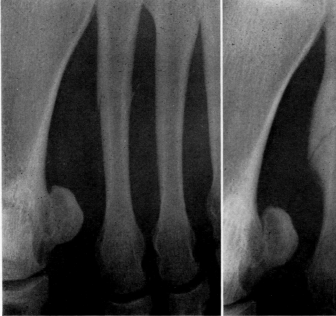
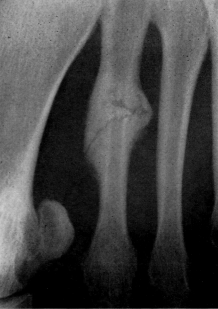

FIG. VIII.29   FIG. VIII.30

A man of 49 had a six weeks history of pain over the forefoot which was swollen and which had been diagnosed as cellulitis and treated with penicillin. The first radiograph shows a small crack across the metatarsal shaft (Fig. VIII.29) but one month later there is to be seen a large amount of callus (Fig. VIII.30), through which the fracture line now extends in the same directions as it did through the shaft.

Despite this, it is not profitable, on clinical grounds, to try and differentiate the various types, as for example in the tibia. Sometimes the early radiological changes show little callus, at other times a large amount. Probably it is the degree of movement that is allowed to occur at the fracture site that is responsible. Figures VIII.29 and VIII.30 show the radiographs of a man who had had pain in his foot for six weeks when the first radiograph (Fig. VIII.29) was taken. The fracture line does not seem very important but after a further month (Fig. VIII.30) the vast amount of callus that occurred can be seen and, interestingly, the fracture lines that were in the cortices have extended, as it were, through the callus in the same directions. This finding indicates that there is still movement at the stress fracture site during healing.

There is some connection between the site of the fracture and the length of history, and the more proximal the fracture is in the metatarsal bone perhaps the longer it is before the symptoms get severe. Figures VIII.31 and VIII.32 show the radiographs of a woman of 57 who had had pain in the foot for eight weeks or so, and the first radiograph shows that there has been a stress fracture at the base of the second metatarsal bone (Fig. VIII.31) which is more clearly seen in the oblique view (Fig. VIII.32). There appears to have been little displacement but even at two months the fracture line can be seen in this patient running straight through the bone, as is usual when the fracture occurs at the base.

Further examples of the difficulty in correlating the natural history of the march fracture to the radiological findings are shown in Figures VIII.33 and VIII.34. The first shows the radiograph of a postman of 51 who had symptoms for six weeks and yet, despite the fracture being at the neck of the second metatarsal bone, it has only caused a small amount of callus and there is no displacement (Fig. VIII.33), whereas the radiograph in Figure VIII.34 shows the foot of a woman of 65 who had only had symptoms for three weeks, which started after she had had a blister on a toe caused by chiropody pads. There was a complete fracture with displacement but which united very quickly.

There is one radiological finding that is important: the second metatarsal bone appears, more often than not, to start a stress fracture in the medial cortex; because many of the usual march fractures start as oblique cracks, as seen in the fibula, which run proximally and laterally, it can be supposed from this that the usual stress is a medial bowing to distract the shaft on that side. This is, however, tenuous and Figures VIII.35 and VIII.36 show in the radiographs an oblique crack in the lateral cortex of the neck of the second metatarsal bone. Perhaps this particular stress fracture was influenced in its site by the osteoarthritis of the adjacent first metatarsophalangeal joint causing the patient to walk on the outer border of her foot.

Stress Fractures of the Third Metatarsal Bone

Stress fractures of the third metatarsal bone are common, but less common than those of the second metatarsal bone. Again they can occur at most ages and they have a far higher percentage of being involved in multiple stress fractures of the metatarsal bones than does the second. One out of every two patients with a stress fracture of the third metatarsal bone will have one or more other metatarsal stress fractures. This characteristic is shared to an even greater extent by the fourth metatarsal, which is more often involved with another metatarsal than it is singly, but usually the other metatarsals involved are either the second or the third. In other words, the first and the

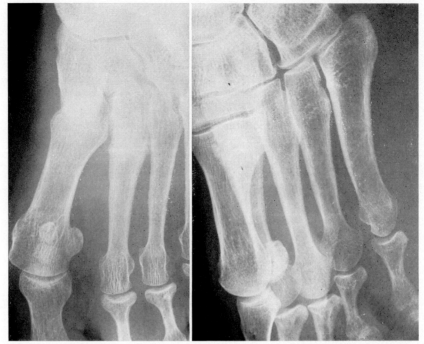

FIG. VIII.31   FIG. VIII.32

A woman of 57 had some eight weeks pain in the forefoot, which eventually brought her to hospital where the radiograph showed that there was a stress fracture at the base of the second metatarsal bone (Fig. VIII.31). The fracture line is more clearly seen in the oblique view (Fig. VIII.32).

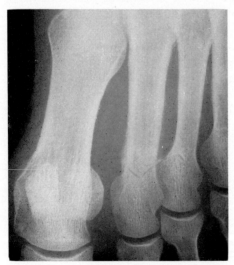

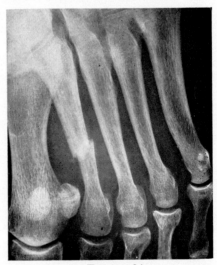

FIG. VIII.33   FIG. VIII.34

A postman of 51 had had pain in his left foot which had been present for six weeks. Although the stress fracture is in the neck of the second metatarsal bone where the stress must be considerable, it has not displaced and there is only a very small amount of callus.

A woman of 65 had pain in her left foot for three weeks after she had had a blister caused by chiropody pads. She had a complete fracture across the shaft with some displacement but little pain. The stress fracture healed quickly.

fifth metatarsals do not share in this multiplicity of fractures and if the fifth metatarsal does in fact share, it is not at its base but in the shaft in which the fracture occurs.

SYMPTOMS AND SIGNS

The history and clinical findings are almost identical for a stress fracture of the third metatarsal bone to that in the second with the exception of the site of pain, tenderness, and swelling when it is found locally, which is over the third metatarsal bone. Figures VIII.37 to VIII.39 show the radiographs of a man of 75 who developed sudden pain in the right foot while walking. Five days later the first radiograph showed no abnormality (Fig. VIII.37) but two weeks later there is to be seen a displaced fracture of the middle of the third metatarsal shaft (Fig. VIII.38), and after a further six weeks it had united soundly (Fig. VIII.39).

RADIOLOGY

There is nothing very special to be noted in the radiographs of stress fractures of the third metatarsal bone that is different from the condition in the adjacent second metatarsal bone. The stress fracture probably starts in the medial cortex; it may displace (Fig. VIII.39) or it may show as simple new bone formation under the periosteum (Fig. VIII.40).

Stress Fractures of the Fourth Metatarsal Bone

Stress fractures of the fourth metatarsal bone are comparatively rare and more often than not are associated with some other metatarsal fracture, usually the second and third. That shown in the radiograph in Figure VIII.41 was in a stout woman of 76 who had had sudden pain and swelling on the outer aspect of the right foot one month before being seen.

Stress Fractures of the Fifth Metatarsal Bone

Stress fractures of the fifth metatarsal are of two types. There is the stress fracture at the base in which a fracture line opens on the lateral side and runs transversely across the bone, often being complete; this is the common sort and occurs next in frequency to the second and third metatarsal stress fractures. Much more rarely there is a stress fracture of the shaft in the same pattern as those in the other metatarsal shafts, but which occur in conjunction with other metatarsal stress fractures.

Figure VIII.42 is the radiograph of a typical stress fracture in the fifth metatarsal base in a man with rheumatoid arthritis treated by steroids. Previously he had had a compression stress fracture of the lower tibia. This figure shows the early appearance of the fracture when there is no displacement or gap at the fracture.

SYMPTOMS AND SIGNS

Pain, worse with activity, is felt on the outer border of the foot. Pain, tenderness and swelling, apart from the site, follow the same course as in other metatarsal stress fractures but may be very much prolonged, as it was in the patient whose radiographs are shown in Figures VIII.43 to VIII.44: the long-standing stress fracture seen in the metatarsal base had started with sudden pain shortly before his first radiograph (Fig. VIII.43) was taken; he was treated in plaster for one month because it was thought the fracture was complete, as indeed it turned out to be. After this he was so much better

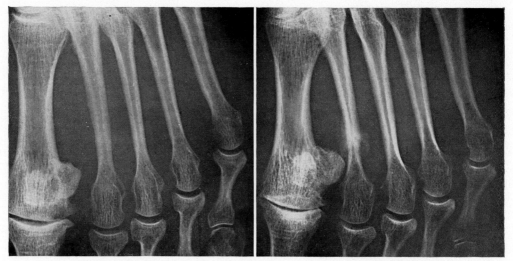

FIG. VIII.35   FIG. VIII.36

A woman of 57 was normal in the morning but in the evening she had considerable pain in her left foot. She had put on weight. She also had osteoarthritis of the first metatarsophalangeal joint. The radiograph in Figure VIII.35, taken when she presented a few days after the pain, shows, when examined carefully, a minute stress fracture on the lateral border of the metatarsal neck rather than in the usual position on the medial side. This may perhaps be an association with the osteoarthritis causing the patient to walk on the lateral side of the foot. Five weeks later the fracture is obvious (Fig. VIII.36).

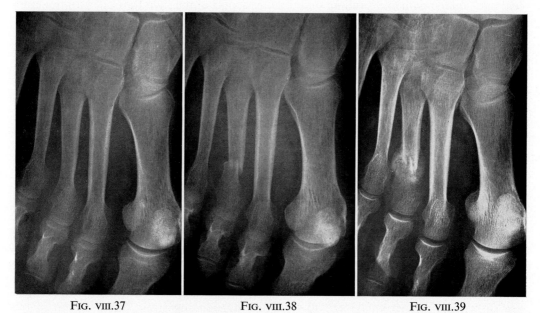

FIG. VIII.37   FIG. VIII.38   FIG. VIII.39

A man of 75 was walking along a road when he felt a sudden pain in his right foot. Five days after the onset of this pain the radiograph in Figure VIII.37 was normal but two weeks later (Fig. VIII.38) there was a stress fracture in the third metatarsal shaft, both obvious and displaced. He had sound union after a further six weeks (Fig. VIII.39).

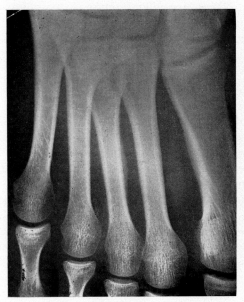

FIG. VIII.40

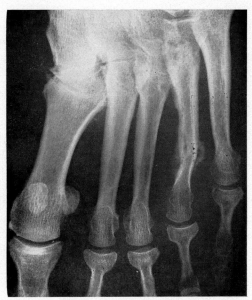

FIG. VIII.41

FIG. VIII.40 An athlete of 19, who had had a stress fracture of the fibula in the past, complained of one week's pain in the right forefoot. A radiograph showed the early haze of new bone formation on both medial and lateral cortex of the third metatarsal shaft at its centre.

FIG.VIII. 41 A stout woman of 76 developed sudden pain and swelling over the outer aspect of the right foot one month before being seen, although there was no localised tenderness at any particular point. The radiograph shows a stress fracture of the fourth metatarsal shaft with angulation and early callus formation.

FIG. VIII.42 A man of 57, a patient with long-standing rheumatoid arthritis treated by steroids, had previously had a compression stress fracture of the lower end of his left tibia. He wore a plastic support on his right knee. He complained of some pain in his right foot. The stress fracture of the base of the fifth metatarsal bone is seen as a thin fracture line which later will show as an obvious transverse crack, as in Figure VIII.43.

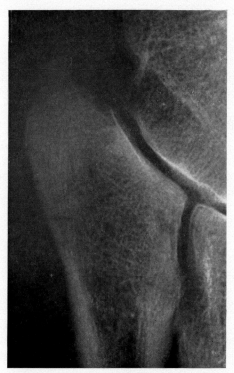

FIG. VIII.42

that he was allowed to go free, only to return with a similar fracture in the opposite fifth metatarsal base. This healed satisfactorily but after two months had passed he returned with more pain in the left foot, and the radiograph (Fig. VIII.44) shows the stress fracture with little sign of union. He was admitted for a bone graft and the lack of union was confirmed at operation.

RADIOLOGY

The radiographs in Figures VIII.42 to VIII.44 show the appearance of a simple stress fracture of the fifth metatarsal base. This appearance, from the thin undisplaced crack in Figure VIII.42 to the established fracture in Figure VIII.43, is quite typical and is comparable to the avulsion of the metatarsal base by injury. The heaping up of the outer lip of the fracture is similar to that seen in transverse stress fractures of the tibial shaft and is an indication that, despite callus formation, healing is not taking place because there is still movement at the fracture site. That this can, in fact, prevent union is shown by the subsequent course of the patient (Fig. VIII.44).

The stress fracture in the shaft of the fifth metatarsal bone is of the same pattern as in the other metatarsal bones but occurs in association with other metatarsal stress fractures.

Stress Fractures of the First Metatarsal Bone

Stress fractures of the first metatarsal are extremely rare and only two examples have been seen. They occur at the first metatarsal base and they are of the compression type, which is not surprising because of the large proportion of the weight that goes through this bone and which, with activity, must be resisted by strong muscular pull.

SYMPTOMS AND SIGNS

Pain with activity is present which gets worse as the activity is continued. There is pain localised to the medial border of the foot with tenderness in the proximal part of the first metatarsal shaft.

RADIOLOGY

The radiographs in Figures VIII.45 and VIII.46 show the development of the haze of internal callus at the first metatarsal base which is very like that seen in the calcaneal stress fracture—which is also compression in type. Displacement of the stress fracture has not been seen.

Multiple Stress Fractures of the Metatarsal Bones

Several metatarsal bones may be affected by stress fractures either at the same time or in sequence. They occur from childhood to old age, in athletes, and in the slim and in the obese. Neither the sex nor the side has any effect on the occurrence.

SYMPTOMS AND SIGNS

Initially the history is the same but it becomes more drawn out and usually the symptoms become more severe than with a single stress fracture although in some patients the course of the condition is as rapid as with a single fracture. The site of the pain is not necessarily felt in more than one place, but tenderness will be found localised

Figs. VIII.43 to VIII.44   A lad of 18, who fenced, complained of sudden pain in his left foot whilst standing and, coming soon to hospital, was treated in a plaster for a month for the stress fracture of the base of the fifth metatarsal bone. This, when first seen as in Figure VIII.43, was already complete but had been present for some while because of the pouting appearance of the transverse crack. When he came out of plaster he still had some tenderness but he was allowed to continue walking, and he then developed a similar fracture in the right fifth metatarsal base. Two months later he returned with more pain in his left foot and the fracture showed no signs of union (Fig. VIII.44). He was admitted to hospital and subjected to bone grafting. At operation the fracture showed non-union.

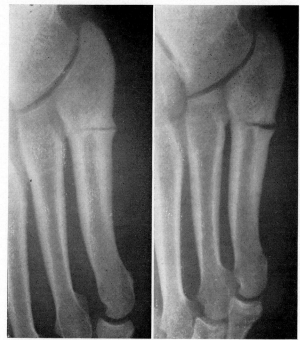

FIG. VIII.43   FIG. VIII.44

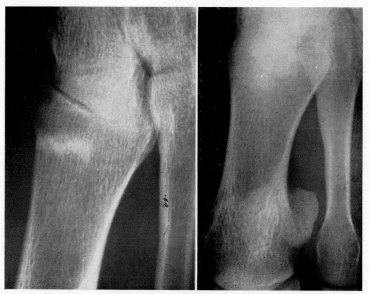

FIG. VIII.45   FIG. VIII.46

A girl of 20, who did a milk-round pushing a float through the streets, developed an aching pain on the inner border of her right foot, which was localised to the base of the first metatarsal bone. The pain was worse walking and relieved by rest. She was tender at the site of the fracture which can be seen to be a compression stress fracture at the base of the first metatarsal bone (Fig. VIII.45). Three months later the internal callus is disappearing (Fig. VIII.46).

to the parts with stress fractures. Swelling, when present, can be greater than with a single stress fracture; in the older patient the whole foot and ankle can become swollen.

RADIOLOGY

A good example of a double stress fracture far distally in the necks of the third and fourth metatarsal bones is shown in Figures VIII.47 and VIII.48; these are the radiographs of a boy of 14 who for three weeks had had pain in his forefoot. He had been sent to the hospital by his doctor with a diagnosis of a march fracture. The radiograph (Fig. VIII.47) showed the two stress fractures, with a haze of internal callus which is much like that of a compression stress fracture, at the junction of the neck with the head of the second and third metatarsal bones. That this appearance was not fortuitous is shown by the further radiograph (Fig. VIII.48) taken a year later. His symptoms subsided within a few months. Had this compression fracture been more distally it would have caused a Freiberg's infraction, or avascular necrosis, of the metatarsal head.

Multiple stress fractures of the metatarsal bones have a very variable radiological appearance. Figure VIII.49 shows the stress fracture in the second metatarsal shaft of a woman of 52 who had had pain for eight months. In this view the callus has obviously organised and continued to expand in an attempt to unite the fracture, but movement at the fracture site has kept open a continuation of the fracture line in the very large amount of callus that has been laid down. The adjacent third metatarsal has also developed a stress fracture, which is at a much earlier stage.

There is a definite sequence in which the metatarsal bones are affected by stress fractures, and the radiograph in Figure VIII.50, which is of a boy of 16, should be compared with the adjacent radiograph in Figure VIII.49. The stress fractures occur in the more medial metatarsal bone first and then in the more lateral one. The same sequence is shown in Figures VIII.51 to VIII.53 in which the stress fractures may follow one on another. The girl in this case was 16 and was thoroughly investigated because of the strange progress of the stress fractures which occurred first in the base of the third right metatarsal bone (Fig. VIII.51) and two months later in the base of the fourth metatarsal bone (Fig. VIII.52) and eight months later in the lower part of the fifth metatarsal shaft and, finally, in the fifth metatarsal base but in an unusual situation with the fracture line medially (Fig. VIII.52).

March fractures can be bilateral but not usually at the same time. The radiographs of a woman of 59 shown in Figures VIII.54 and VIII.55 show stress fractures of the second and third metatarsal shafts of the left foot, in which there was a hallux valgus, and, 15 months later, the stress fracture in the fourth metatarsal of the right foot.

DIAGNOSIS OF MARCH FRACTURES

Being the best known of all stress fractures the diagnosis is very often considered in any painful condition of the forefoot especially when it is associated with increased or unusual activity. Again radiological confirmation is often present when the first radiograph is taken although it can be delayed over several weeks.

Other conditions of the foot which may be obvious, such as a hallux rigidus, may, by their very prominence, confuse because of a cursory enquiry into the history followed by a superficial examination. On the other hand conditions such as gout can mislead even the most experienced, and it can co-exist, as can rheumatoid arthritis, when a 'flare up' may be held responsible for the symptoms. The blanket diagnosis of meta-

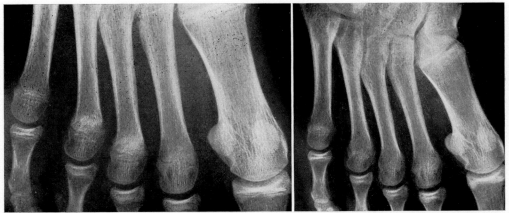

<table>
<tr><td>FIG. VIII.47</td><td>FIG. VIII.48</td></tr>
</table>

A boy of 14 had a three weeks history of pain in the forefoot and the radiographs show compression stress fractures of the necks of the third and fourth metatarsal bones. That this appearance is not merely chance is shown by the follow-up radiograph a year later, where the haze of internal callus has disappeared and sound union occurred. This is the sort of fracture which a little farther down into the head would cause an avascular necrosis.

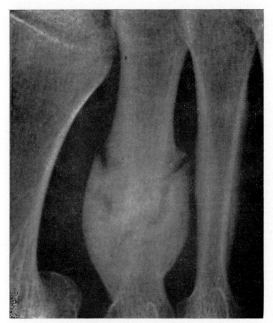

FIG. VIII.49

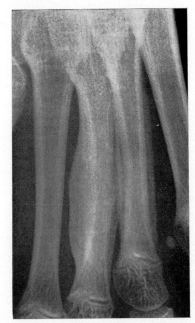

FIG. VIII.50

A woman of 52 had pain in her left forefoot for eight months. The radiograph shows quite clearly a well-developed stress fracture of the second metatarsal bone which has tried to unite, but the fracture line persists through the well-organised callus. The stress fracture of the third metatarsal shaft might easily be missed in the original radiograph. It was probably a long thin fracture to give this amount of callus.

A boy of 16 had had two weeks swelling in his foot but no injury and the pain made him seek attention. He has a stress fracture of the third metatarsal bone on the left foot, which has healed well, but he also has an earlier fracture of the fourth metatarsal bone. These fractures are comparable to those of the woman of 52 in Figure VIII.49.

M

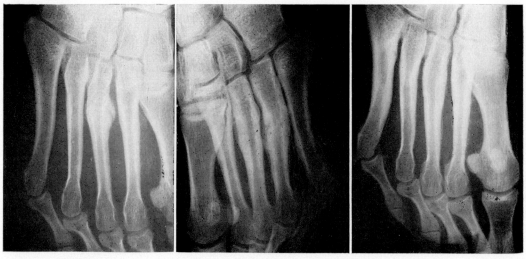

FIG. VIII.51   FIG. VIII.52   FIG. VIII.53

A girl of 16 had sustained a stress fracture of the base of her third metatarsal bone (Fig. VIII.51). Two months later she developed a stress fracture in her fourth metatarsal bone, again near the base (Fig. VIII.52). Eight months after that the fifth metatarsal was shown to have had a fracture transversely in its medial cortex at the base, which is unusual. In retrospect it was observed that the shaft of the fifth metatarsal had also had a stress fracture which had healed (Fig. VIII.53). She was investigated very fully for her general condition but no abnormalities were to be found.

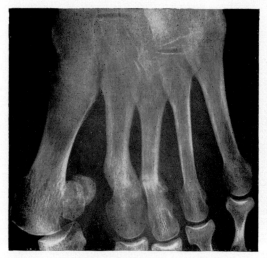 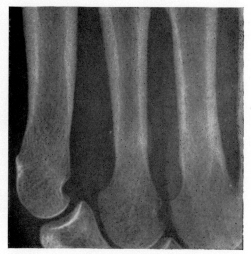

FIG. VIII.54   FIG. VIII.55

A woman of 59 had had pain in the left foot which went into the third left toe the year previously. She was now complaining of pain in the right forefoot. The radiographs show that she had had stress fractures of the second and third metatarsal bones the previous year, but that in the right foot she had a new stress fracture of the fourth metatarsal shaft near the neck. Bilateral march fractures are uncommon at the same time, because one side initiates inactivity which prevents the opposite side developing.

tarsalgia—although literally true—may lead to entirely useless, if not wrong, treatment. All the other forms of foot strain may be inculpated and all can be discarded by the full and careful general appreciation of the localised symptoms and signs.

TREATMENT

Simple support is sufficient in almost all march fractures, with sufficient restraint on activity to allow the fracture to heal. If elastic adhesive strapping or any other form of firm binding is used, it must of course be applied from the base of the toes so that the metatarsal bones are firmly gripped from the heads and thereby obtain a measure of immobilisation both from the binding and the adjacent bones.

For the patient with severe symptoms which persist despite simple measures, a wellfitting plaster cast to below the knee allows the patient to walk without pain; even this at times does not allow sufficient immobilisation to obtain healing, as was the case with the patient in Figures VIII.43 to VIII.44.

Supports of various kinds in the shoes are not very helpful in general, but a shoe giving firm support and with a soft sole is good; in women attention to the height of the heel may also be necessary because a high heel, forward sloping, may allow excess strain to occur in the metatarsal bone affected with an increase in pain. In general a shoe giving comfort to the patient is satisfactory.

Stress Fractures of the Sesamoid Bones of the Hallux

The problem of a stress fracture in a sesamoid bone is a difficult one because many of them are bipartite; however, there is little doubt that some of these at least become bipartite through a stress fracture which fails to heal. That a child should get a painful forefoot which remains painful for only a week or two and which does not cause serious trouble, except perhaps to restrict activity slightly, is often the only history and it is only by very careful examination and radiography that the stress fractures can be proven. Added to this the sesamoid stress fracture is not at all common. It has not been seen in adults.

The child who complains of pain in the forefoot will often have noticed the pain to start or to be worse on jumping and landing on the forefoot. This history suggests a contusion and with expectant treatment the child gets better. No fracture may be seen in the initial radiograph and the true diagnosis will not be made. Only by careful observation and follow-up radiographs can there be any certainty of the diagnosis, which is also difficult because if there is a stress fracture in the sesamoid bone visible in the radiograph it may be thought that this was a bipartite bone and the diagnosis of a contusion upheld.

Careful examination will localise the pain absolutely to the affected sesamoid; serial radiography will confirm the diagnosis, as was the case of the girl whose radiographs are shown in Figures VIII.56 to VIII.58. At first she was thought to have a bipartite medial sesamoid bone of the left foot but the tangential view (Fig. VIII.57) shows a difference in the texture of the medial and the lateral sesamoid bones caused by callus formation within the bone. Nearly three months later the difference was no longer present.

Figures VIII.59 and VIII.60 are the radiographs of the medial sesamoid of another girl, in which the initial radiograph (Fig. VIII.59) shows a small gap between the proximal

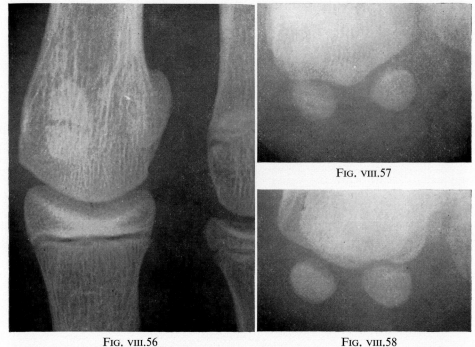

FIG. VIII.56   FIG. VIII.58

FIG. VIII.57

A girl of 11 developed pain in the left forefoot over the medial sesamoid of the hallux which remained painful for a month, having been treated in a stiff bandage followed by a plaster. The original radiographs showed a crack through the medial sesamoid, and in Figure VIII.57 three weeks later there is some change in the bone texture which has left the medial sesamoid slightly denser than the lateral. Three months later the increased density of the medial sesamoid has disappeared (Fig. VIII.58).

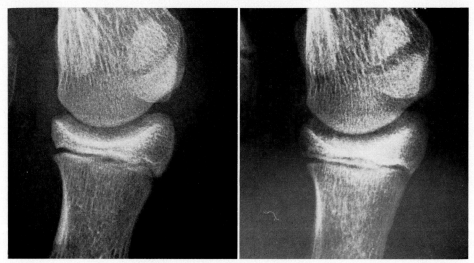

FIG. VIII.59   FIG. VIII.60

A girl of 12 developed a swollen and painful first metatarsophalangeal joint of the right foot. Her history included a bang on the heel only about six weeks previously but she had not injured the front of the foot. Clinically the medial sesamoid was extremely tender and the first radiograph showed a sesamoid which had a small gap and might well have been bipartite but for the clinical findings (Fig. VIII.59). One month later the gap is larger (Fig. VIII.60).

and distal poles of the medial sesamoid but three months later, with a very similar radiographic projection, the gap has increased (Fig. VIII.60). The first radiograph of the sesamoid was taken very soon after the typical symptoms had begun and the sesamoid having broken, the parts were distracted. This lesion is comparable to those seen in the patella.

Because of the difficulty of lateral tangential views in the radiography of the sesamoids it is very difficult ever to get a picture of the stress fracture before separation occurs.

The treatment of the condition is basically expectant because the child recovers fully and quickly. Simple supportive measures, such as strapping, a padded shoe and slight restriction of activity are sufficient and even though the fracture does not unite it appears to give no symptoms in later life.

CHAPTER NINE

STRESS FRACTURES OF THE UPPER LIMB AND TRUNK

Stress fractures have been seen in the arm in the humerus and ulna, but they have not been seen in the radius. In the shoulder girdle the clavicle can have a stress fracture but none has been seen in the scapula other than after radiotherapy. The first rib has a very definite stress fracture of its own quite apart from the 'silent' stress fracture at its anterior end.

In the trunk the ribs used to have many stress fractures because they often occurred after thoracoplasty and were secondary to the deformity that had been produced; but there are several groups of people in whom stress fractures occur in the ribs and, if they are not understood, may prove a great disability to the patient. Athletes get stress fractures of the ribs on the side of the dominant arm used in such sports as tennis, and mostly in the upper ribs. Pregnancy can cause stress fractures of a rib—again perhaps from 'deformity' but this must be considered physiological—and rheumatoid arthritis and irradiation treatment can predispose to a type of stress fracture in the ribs.

Stress fractures in the spine have not been seen, with the exception of spondylolisthesis of the lower lumbar region. There is considerable difference of opinion about the cause of the acquired spondylolisthesis in the adolescent but one cause quite definitely is a stress fracture in or near the pars interarticularis. Stress fractures of the pelvis have already been dealt with in Chapter Five.

Stress Fractures of the Humerus

Stress fractures of the humerus are seen particularly in adolescents or young adults who do much throwing or use the arm a great deal. Probably many are misdiagnosed as muscle violence fractures, as might well be expected because of the rather dramatic events that can take place, as was the case in the patient in Figures IX.1 to IX.5. Had not the practitioner spent considerable time and care in taking the history it might not have been realised that this was a stress fracture.

SYMPTOMS AND SIGNS

After a period of activity in throwing or similar use of the arm an ache begins to be noticed, particularly after the sport is over, and then gradually it comes on during sport. It also may be noticed if feverish activity is undertaken for a short time, when the arm will feel tired. The pain may be referred downwards from the upper arm to the elbow and even the forearm. Examination of the arm will reveal tenderness around the shaft of the humerus but there will be full movements of the shoulder and elbow, provided, of course, the stress fracture has not become complete. The patient in Figures IX.1 to IX.5 broke the arm when actually throwing although there was excellent clinical

174

FIGS. IX.1 to IX.5 A boy of 15 developed pain in his right arm over some weeks playing cricket, particularly when he was doing a lot of throwing practice. It always ached after this but never if he did not practice throwing; he was right-handed. The day before being seen he threw the ball to another player, the arm gave a loud snap and fell useless to his side. Further questioning revealed that the arm ached after any particular activity in which it was greatly used such as bowling. The radiograph when the patient was first seen showed a long spiral crack (Fig. IX.1). The enlarged view of the upper humerus (Fig. IX.2) shows an apparent erosion around the medial cortex just below the neck, with some subperiosteal callus already present. Serial views showed progressive healing of the forearm (Figs. IX.3 and IX.4) and one year later it was quite normal (Fig. IX.5).

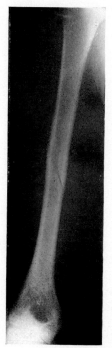
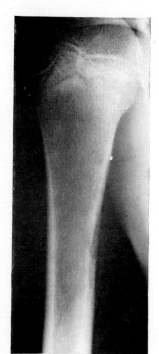

FIG. IX.1   FIG. IX.2

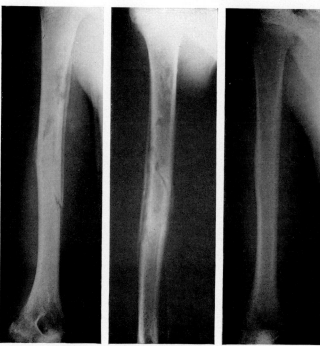

FIG. IX.3   FIG. IX.4   FIG. IX.5

and radiological evidence that a stress fracture had pre-existed for some time. At the time of his examination all the signs were those of a fractured shaft of the humerus. A similar fracture but lower in the shaft is shown in Figure IX.6, which is the radiograph of the humerus of a boy of 15 who was left-handed and who felt a very severe pain on throwing a cricket ball. Before that he had on occasions after playing cricket felt an ache in the arm but he had had no stiffness or other disability before the acute episode when the fracture became complete.

RADIOLOGY

The early lesion in the humerus can easily be missed unless particular care is taken in getting good views of the shaft to show the earliest changes. Figures IX.7 to IX.9 show the humerus of a boy of 15 who had been on holiday. During that time he had done much throwing and when he returned home he did a lot of wall painting. Later he developed cramp in his hand when writing. The pain was always localised, apart from this, to the proximal part of the arm and clinically he was tender around the upper humeral shaft. The radiograph showed an area which, when compared to that in Figure IX.2, was easily seen to be an early stress fracture of the medial cortex of the humerus so that the diagnosis was made with confidence. However, the rather peculiar erosion and roughening of the medial cortex might easily be mistaken for a normal variant of the upper end of the humerus or 'periostitis'. In Figure IX.7 it is just possible to see the crack through the medial cortex but in the second radiograph, some four weeks later, the lesion, although healing, shows the stress fracture perhaps better. Three months later, in Figure IX.9, healing is almost complete.

DIAGNOSIS

This is easy provided the usual criteria of pain after exercise and the finding of local tenderness in the shaft of the humerus are understood. Radiologically confirmation has always been present in those cases seen. Because the humerus is not weight-bearing and because the stresses that caused the fracture are intermittent, the course can be lengthy so a history of two or three months should not deter the clinician from suspecting this stress fracture.

When a youth attends with a fractured shaft of humerus with a history of 'muscle violence'—that is, that he was throwing a ball hard when his arm broke—careful enquiry for pain preceding this must be made, otherwise the diagnosis will not be made and the radiological confirmation of the pre-existing lesion may not be seen.

TREATMENT

If the arm has a complete fracture it is treated by the usual methods. If the fracture is not complete, rest from those activities that cause pain is sufficient. This was the only treatment given to the patient whose radiographs are shown in Figures IX.7 to IX.9 and he was entirely better within a few weeks.

DISCUSSION

The finding of stress fractures of the humerus at about the age of 15 in boys is probably fortuitous and it is likely that other examples could occur at an earlier or later age; particularly ought they to be seen in athletes practising throwing energetically to improve their speed or distance. Although cricket has been inculpated as the sport,

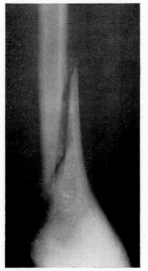

FIG. IX.6   A boy of 15 broke his left arm throwing a cricket ball. He had had, on occasions, and usually after playing cricket, an ache in the left arm before the moment when he threw the ball and the arm broke. He had no stiffness in the arm before this and he was left-handed. The radiograph taken immediately afterwards showed a spiral fracture with callus. Four weeks later when this radiograph was taken there was union. This was undoubtedly a stress fracture which broke completely.

FIG. IX.6

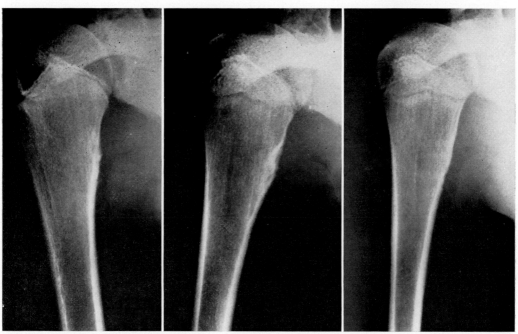

FIG. IX.7   FIG. IX.8   FIG. IX.9

A boy of 15 developed pain in his right arm after a holiday in which he did a lot of throwing. After this he did a lot of wall painting and the pain would gradually come on while he was doing this. He found that he had cramp in his hand if he did much writing. The pain he felt in the arm was localised to the upper end of the humerus. The radiograph showed a rough area of the medial cortex of the humerus just at its neck and an irregular line through the medial cortex and possibly running down the shaft from that level (Fig. IX.7). The symptoms were so typical of a stress lesion that this was diagnosed and a further radiograph a month later showed slight improvement but the stress fracture in the medial cortex is now more clear. Three months later the radiograph showed healing (Fig. IX.9). He had no further symptoms.

in two out of the three examples given here it was not bowling that produced the stress but throwing in fielding practice that caused symptoms.

Stress Fractures of the Ulna

Stress fractures of the ulna occur in the olecranon as the classical javelin thrower's elbow (Figs. IX.10 to IX.12) and in the shaft or lower part of the ulna, often in those unfortunate enough to be confined to a self-propelled wheelchair (Figs. IX.15 to IX.17).

SYMPTOMS AND SIGNS

The javelin thrower exerts a tremendous thrust when throwing with full extension of the elbow. Gradually an ache occurs after throwing and then during throwing until the sport has to be stopped. With a little rest symptoms improve and the throwing started again only to produce more symptoms.

Examination reveals only local tenderness which is at and around the olecranon. Care must be taken to exclude the many avulsions that can be caused around the elbow with this sport—and which later show as small flakes or exostoses around the joint (Figs. IX.13 and IX.14).

Symptoms from an ulna shaft in which a stress fracture is developing are, as is usual, pain after use and later pain during use (Figs. IX.18 and IX.19). The pain may be felt in the wrist or hand: rotating the forearm may cause pain as does propelling the wheelchair. Finally it is almost impossible to use the forearm for any except the lightest activity.

Clinical examination will reveal tenderness localised to that part of the ulna affected which is usually in the distal two thirds of the shaft.

RADIOLOGY

The early radiological signs in the ulna can be difficult to see (Figs. IX.20 to IX.21) but in other cases it is obvious as in Figures IX.15 to IX.17; but even in this patient the callus that pre-existed the complete fracture can be seen easily.

TREATMENT

Treatment of a stress fracture of the ulna in the athlete is difficult because without rest from sport for a long time healing will not take place; fortunately, at least for the amateur, healing by fibrous union can occur in the olecranon and be satisfactory. A plaster cast from axilla to wrist is necessary to ensure complete rest. Probably internal fixation could be used equally well. Stress fractures in the shaft of the ulna respond rapidly to immobilisation in a plaster cast.

Stress Fractures of the Clavicle

It is very rare for the clavicle to have a stress fracture and only one has been seen— in a man whose radiograph is shown in Figures IX.22 and IX.23. This patient was accustomed to fill a coal-scuttle as a routine and in a certain way and one evening he developed pain in the right shoulder. Two days later it was so severe that he had to attend hospital. He was quite certain there had been no injury or violence to the shoulder. Two months later he had good union. Although the history is short, there

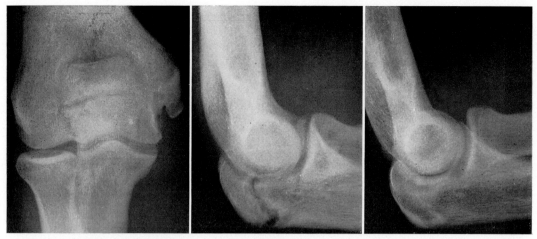

| FIG. IX.10 | FIG. IX.11 | FIG. IX.12 |

A keen javelin thrower of 16 complained of pain in his right elbow for four weeks. He had no pain on the inner side of the elbow at the medial epicondyle. He threw his javelin with the usual clockwise spin. The radiographs show a stress fracture of the olecranon. This is not an unusual epiphysis and the normal left elbow is shown in Figure IX.12. Such fractures can be difficult to unite but fibrous union can be satisfactory in some patients. The anteroposterior view (Fig. IX.10) also shows the damage to the medial epicondyle that is often seen with this sport.

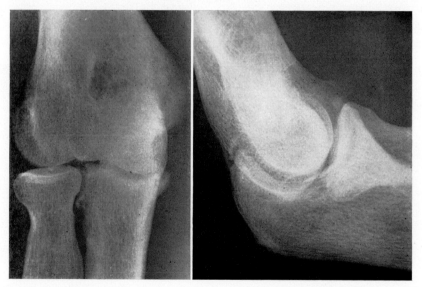

| FIG. IX.13 | FIG. IX.14 |

These radiographs show the end results of javelin throwing. A middle-aged man attended with a history of having wrenched his elbow two weeks previously while starting a car. He said that in his youth he had been an enthusiastic javelin thrower. When seen, his elbow had already regained full movements and he had no symptoms but the radiographs show the considerable damage that can occur, particularly to the upper ulna, from the strain of the throwing; in his case, the humerus has escaped with little damage around the medial epicondyle.

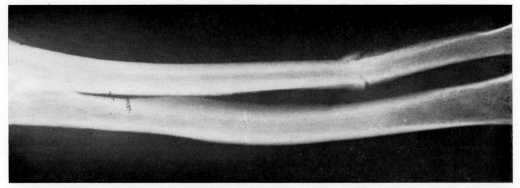

FIG. IX.15

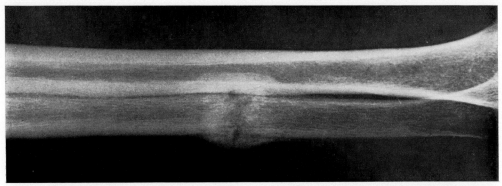

FIG. IX.16

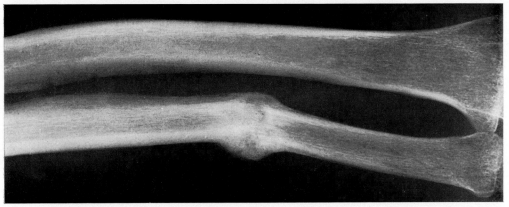

FIG. IX.17

A woman of 51 sustained a fracture of the shaft of the right humerus. She also suffered from disseminated sclerosis and had led a wheelchair existence for several years. Union in the humerus was slow and needed internal fixation. While undergoing extreme efforts at rehabilitation the patient exercised her left arm by rotating a 'ship's wheel' loaded to give resistance. She used her left arm with such energy that she gradually got pain in the forearm. She was found to be acutely tender over the ulna, and the subsequent radiographs showed a stress fracture and the healing thereof. The first radiograph in Figure IX.15 shows that the fracture became complete but that there was pre-existing callus. Figures IX.16 and IX.17 show the subsequent course.

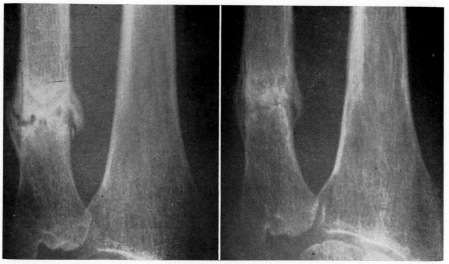

FIG. ix.18   FIG. ix.19

A middle-aged hospital matron had pain in the left forearm for eight weeks but had had no injury and had been treated on and off in a splint during that time. Investigation showed no evidence of serious osteoporosis and all her blood tests were normal. The radiographs show the progress of the stress fracture. Once it was properly immobilised after the first radiograph (Fig. ix.18) healing was rapid (Fig. ix.19).

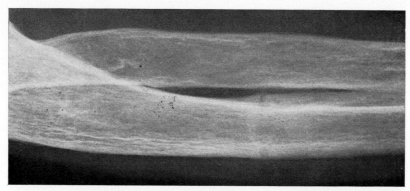

FIG. ix.20

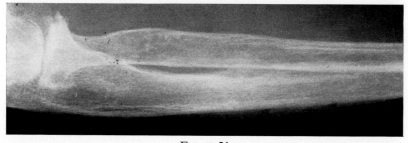

FIG. ix.21

A retired hospital matron of 84 fractured the neck of her left femur for which a Thompson prosthesis was cemented in place. She returned to full function but later arthritis of the knees caused her to use a wheelchair. She was generally osteoporotic. The right ulna developed a stress fracture from the unaccustomed wheeling of her chair. The initial radiograph (Fig. ix.20) shows the stress fracture to be complete but without displacement.

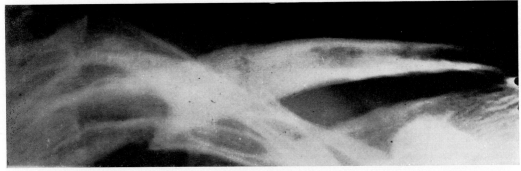

FIG. IX.22

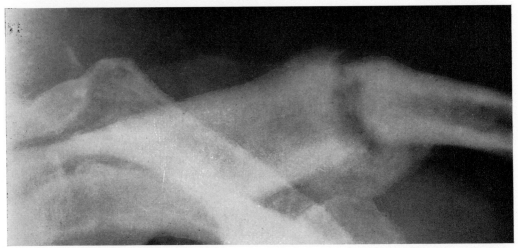

FIG. IX.23

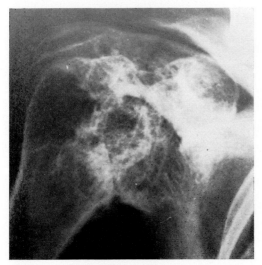

FIG. IX.24

FIGS. IX.22 and IX.23 A man who was accustomed to fill coal-scuttles developed pain in his right shoulder. Two days later the pain was so severe that he attended hospital where he was found to have a stress fracture of the clavicle. He was absolutely certain that there was no injury or muscle violence. The first radiograph in Figure IX.22 shows the fracture line with a haze of callus and two months later that there is union with slight angulation (Fig. IX.23).

FIG. IX.24 A woman of 50 had had radiotherapy in high dosage for a carcinoma of the breast. The bones near the shoulder have become osteoporotic as a result. The acromion has sustained a type of stress fracture secondary to the osteoporosis but the symptoms were typical of a stress fracture.

is too much callus at the fracture site to have occurred in two days so the stress fracture must have started some time previously.

Stress Fractures of the Scapula

These have not been seen in normal patients but they were seen, and perhaps still are, in those unfortunate patients who have had deep x-ray treatment near the shoulder after carcinoma of the breast. Figure IX.24 shows a fracture of the acromion which had all the signs and symptoms of a stress fracture in a patient who had had much deep x-ray therapy for a carcinoma of the breast. Although this is a pathological fracture it will give the same symptoms as a stress fracture.

Stress Fractures of the Ribs

Stress fractures of the ribs were extremely common after thoracoplasty, which operation is now rarely done. Stress fractures of the ribs are seen in athletes, particularly those who play tennis or similar games, in pregnant women, and in patients on steroids or who have had radiotherapy.

In the first rib a stress fracture can cause severe symptoms in the arm and, unless this is realised, the examination may not elicit the localised tenderness. Figure IX.25 shows an excellent example in a girl of 12. The symptoms, not so typical of a stress fracture, were of very acute pain in the right shoulder and upper arm and in the right side of the neck. She was very tender in the posterior triangle over the stress fracture in the first rib. The symptoms resolved quickly with simple rest from the activities causing the pain.

Figure IX.26 shows the stress fracture in the third rib of a girl of 15, a doctor's daughter, who had had pain in the left shoulder which was first noticed while dressing. However, her shoulder remained painful while playing games and her symptoms lasted for three months. Suddenly they became worse with a wrench and the arm had to be rested. A year later she had a similar sequence of events and the radiographs taken at that time (Fig. IX.26) were misinterpreted as being those of a tumour and a block dissection was done, including the ribs above and below. Normal fracture healing was discovered.

Figure IX.27 shows the radiograph of the eighth rib of an athlete of 19 who noticed pain developing particularly while serving at tennis over a period of five weeks. When not playing tennis he had no pain. He did not attend for advice for a further two months, when he felt a lump at the site of the pain. He had developed a stress fracture of the eighth right rib.

Pregnancy as opposed to chronic bronchitis will produce a true stress fracture caused by the altered stresses on the rib cage by fecundity; it is a true stress fracture because pregnancy is certainly not abnormal to women, even if most of the time it is not usual. Figure IX.28 shows the radiograph of a woman of 37 who developed pain while pregnant; after some while the radiographs confirmed the stress fracture. This appearance is again somewhat suggestive of a neoplasm, but if the signs and symptoms are carefully elicited a true diagnosis on clinical grounds may be made; particularly is this important in the pregnant woman so that radiographs may be avoided.

Steroids, as in the rest of the skeleton, make a patient liable to a type of stress fracture

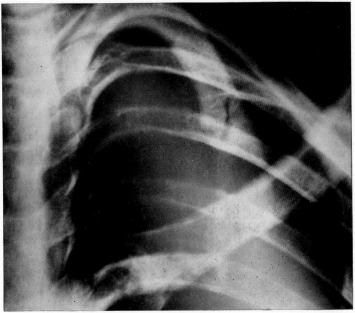

FIG. IX.25

A girl of 12 developed acute pain in the right shoulder and in the right side of the neck. Careful examination, however, revealed that the greatest tenderness was in the posterior triangle over the first rib in which there was a stress fracture.

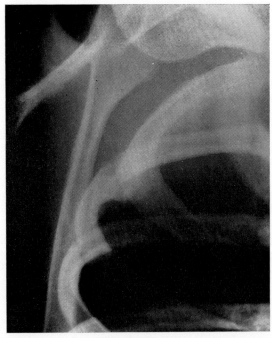

FIG. IX.26

FIG. IX.26   A girl of 15, a doctor's daughter, complained of pain in the left shoulder which started while dressing but got better in two days. Afterwards using the arm or shoulder caused pain. The symptoms lasted three months when a sudden jolt caused extreme pain and she had to rest the arm. She was very active in sports. She was diagnosed as having myositis but one year later reattended with a similar pain in the left shoulder made worse by sport. Some pain occurred in the region of the third rib on certain movements of the shoulder. The stress fracture of the rib was erroneously diagnosed as a tumour and a block excision was done.

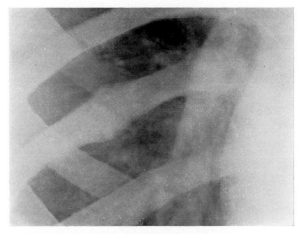

FIG. IX.27

A youth of 19 playing tennis developed pain particularly while serving. He had no pain when not playing tennis. He had had the pain for five weeks but attended two months later because he felt a lump at the site of the pain which was the callus of the stress fracture of the eighth rib. Tennis, perhaps being one of the most common sports using the arm with great vigour, is also the commonest cause of the athlete developing a stress fracture of the rib.

FIG. IX.28

A woman aged 37 towards the end of a normal pregnancy gave a slight cough and felt a pain in the lower chest. It was some months before the radiograph was taken but it still showed a stress fracture of the ninth rib. Such appearances can be very suggestive of infection or even neoplasm. These particular stress fractures in pregnancy are common but do not need to be confirmed radiologically. Treatment may be difficult but the pain will usually subside with time even if the fracture does not unite quickly.

N

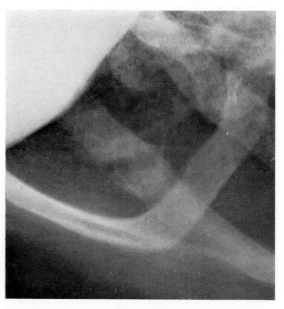

FIG. IX.28

of the rib. Figure IX.29 shows the ribs of a man of 45 who had been taking steroids for rheumatoid arthritis. The diagnosis is easy with so many fractures. Although steroids have predisposed the patient to the fractures they heal quickly and without much trouble. Figure IX.30 shows the type of fracture seen in the radiograph of a rib after deep x-ray treatment. The appearance might be mistaken for a recurrence of the tumour for which the treatment was given, and the symptoms and signs of a slowly progressive pathological fracture are identical to those of a simple stress fracture. However, serial radiography will show improvement in the lesion and clinically the pain also gets better rather than worse.

A cervical rib has been known to develop a stress fracture. Figure IX.31 shows a radiograph of the cervical rib of a woman of 61, excised because it developed a lump with increasing pain. In previous radiographs—unfortunately no longer available—taken before the pain was severe, the cervical rib was intact; after excision the radiograph confirmed a pseudoarthrosis, presumed to be secondary to a stress fracture.

Spondylolisthesis

Spondylolisthesis of Newman's group II is caused, if not always, at least quite often, by a stress fracture of the pars interarticularis.

A study of the symptoms and signs shows that the progress of the condition follows very closely that of a stress fracture elsewhere. Confusion arises, however, because once the stress fracture has become complete across the pars interarticularis it may displace and non-union becomes established. From then on the symptoms of a different condition occur—those of an unstable back.

The common age for the early symptoms and signs of spondylolisthesis is in the early adolescence. Backache, worse with exercise, better with rest, occurs. It is localised to the low lumbar region—rarely higher—and is always associated very clearly with some particular or general activity, from swimming to hurdling. Even to a 10-year-old child this sequence of events is noticeable.

It is at this stage that no radiological confirmation is present. The child is treated as having a strain. Sport is modified, perhaps given up, and ten years later backache again supervenes and an established spondylolisthesis is seen in the radiographs.

The pars interarticularis is not easy to see even in the best radiographs, and it is very difficult to be certain that a small oblique crack in one or other pars does in fact exist. If further radiographs confirm the increasing gap it is by then too late to treat the stress fracture because, even with prolonged immobilisation, union will not occur.

The best treatment will mean that never has it been certain that a spondylolisthesis has existed. Occasionally the unilateral stress fracture of a pars interarticularis is more obvious than usual, and perhaps because it is on one side only will heal more easily than one that was as obvious but bilateral. Figures IX.32 to IX.35 show the radiographs of a girl of 11. The pars interarticularis shown in Figure IX.32 appears to have a definite fracture line in it. With continued immobilisation it healed (Fig. IX.34). The opposite pars is shown reversed for comparison.

If the stress fracture is any more obvious than that seen in the radiograph in Figure IX.32, as it was in Figure IX.36, the radiograph of a boy of 10, failure of conservative treatment is certain and the 'slip' will gradually increase with established non-union (Figs. IX.37 to IX.39).

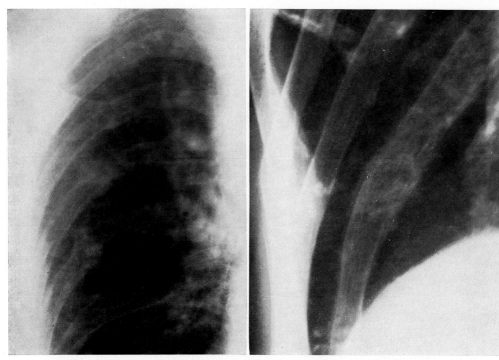

FIG. IX.29

FIG. IX.30

A man of 45 with rheumatoid arthritis treated with steroids developed a series of stress fractures in his ribs. As in other areas, steroid treatment and rheumatoid arthritis both predispose to stress fractures. Here, five or six ribs can be seen to have fractures.

A man of 68 had had a partial excision of the scapula followed by radiotherapy for a solitary plasmacytoma. Two years later he developed insidiously a pain in the ninth rib in the anterior axillary line. The first radiograph showed a fracture difficult to show in a reproduction but six weeks later the uniting stress fracture in the osteoporotic rib secondary to the radiotherapy is clearly seen.

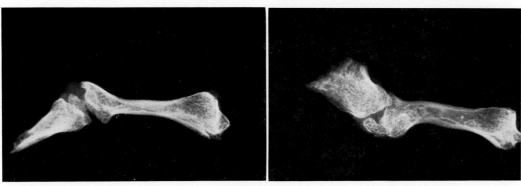

FIG. IX.31

A woman of 61 known to have a cervical rib developed increasing pain and a hard bony mass was felt in the neck. It was thought wise to excise the rib. The radiograph of the specimen showed that there was a pseudoarthrosis where previously there had been a normal cervical rib. Excision is not usually necessary in the treatment of a stress fracture but without doubt this was the correct treatment here.

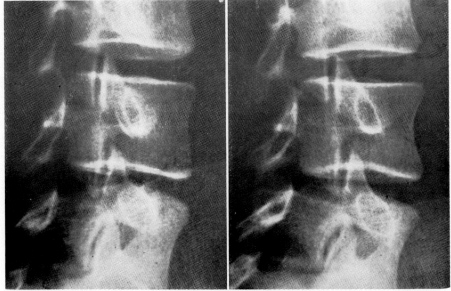

FIG. IX.32   FIG. IX.33

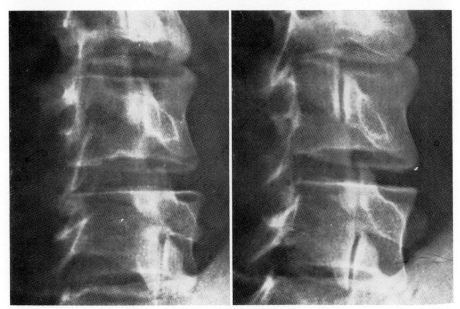

FIG. IX.34   FIG. IX.35

A girl of 11 had a typical backache suggesting spondylolisthesis. It came on with activity, was worse after games and was eased by rest. Oblique radiographs showed that there was a crack in the pars interarticularis on the left in the fourth lumbar vertebra (Fig. IX.32). The right pars interarticularis, shown in Figure IX.33, reversed left to right for comparison, showed no fracture. She was treated in a plaster jacket for nearly a year. Fourteen months after the original radiographs further oblique views show that the stress fracture has disappeared, and united (Fig. IX.34). Figure IX.35 is the radiograph of the right pars interarticularis at the same time, again reversed left to right. Note that in Figure IX.32 the inferior surface of the 'neck' through which the fracture runs is apparently slightly displaced to form a notch and this is more obvious when it is compared to the opposite side. A year later this notch has disappeared.

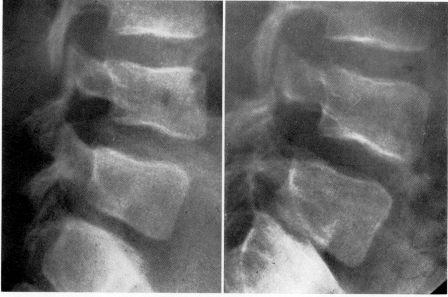

FIG. ix.36   FIG. ix.37

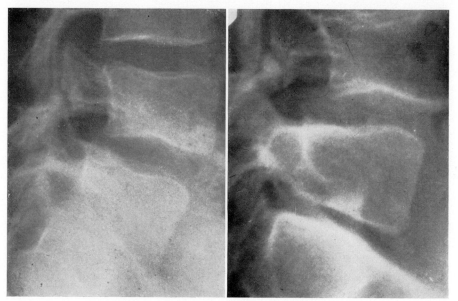

FIG. ix.38   FIG. ix.39

A boy of 10 had a painful back which he said gave way when he was playing football. The radiographs taken suggested that he had already developed a spondylolisthesis and that the fourth lumbar vertebra was slightly forward on the fifth. In the lateral view there was a definite fracture in the pars interarticularis which, although it did not seem so, must have been complete. Despite immobilisation in a jacket the condition progressed inexorably. In Figure ix.37 a year later, the slip has increased, but the fracture line is not much wider. In Figure ix.38, two years after the first radiograph, the slip has again increased and there is sclerosis around the margin of the fracture although the width of the fracture line has decreased. Figure ix.39 is the radiograph six years after he was first seen. He has a well-established spondylolisthesis but some form of healing has been attempted because the gap in the pars interarticularis is no wider and there appears to have been an attempt at filling the gap with new bone, thus elongating the pars interarticularis.

CHAPTER TEN

STRESS AVULSIONS AND OSTEOCHONDRITIS

Introduction

The pattern of stress fractures in children and the adolescent is particularly interesting when studied in the leg. Those stress fractures that occur in the metatarsal bones, the fibula, the tibia and the pubis have been described. The femur has been conspicuous by its absence, and the patella, which shows stress fractures in adolescents, has a different pattern of stress lesions as the age of the child gets younger. It has also been shown that the tibial tubercle can be avulsed in the adolescent.

At different ages different stresses appear to cause different fractures in the child or adolescent, and in this chapter those avulsions in youth that replace certain stress fractures of the adult are discussed, in particular those around the pelvis and the lesser trochanter of the femur and around the knee, particularly in the lower pole of the patella and the tibial tubercle. Despite all these, it will still be realised that there is a gap in the pattern of stress lesions at the age when Perthes' disease of the hip occurs and, later, when slipped upper femoral epiphyses are seen. However, about the same age that each of the latter occur there are pelvic stress lesions; the anterior iliac spines are avulsed at the same age as the upper femoral epiphysis may slip, and stress fractures of the pubis occur shortly after the age of Perthes' disease. The child does not have a stress fracture of the calcaneus; the condition known as Sever's disease is seen instead and is in fact a stress fracture of the apophysis. Most stress fractures of the tibia in children are in the uppermost third, in or near the region of the tibial tubercle, and it is not surprising that there is seen a stress lesion of the tubercle itself which, in the more mature adolescent, has already been seen as an avulsion of the complete tubercle and part of the tibial plateau. Again, at the same age at which the so-called osteochondritis of the tibial tubercle occurs, the lower pole of the patella may also develop a stress lesion. Stress fractures of the navicular bone of the foot have been seen in the adult, and in the child this bone becomes avascular and the condition is called Köhler's disease, which, if not in all, is in many children secondary to a stress fracture within that bone which causes the avascularity.

Studying the natural history of stress fractures leads to the conclusion that the all-important factor in the cause is muscular activity; also that in most stress fractures there is a history of symptoms gradually getting worse with activity. Sometimes the onset of symptoms is sudden but careful examination of the patient and the radiographs will show that the stress fracture has existed before the sudden onset, and quite often such a presentation indicates that a partial stress fracture had become complete. In certain parts of the body in children and adolescents a muscular attachment can be avulsed.

Many bony avulsions are caused by sudden muscle violence but others are true stress fractures through the part that has been avulsed. No such avulsion can be considered a stress avulsion unless there is a clear history of pain associated with activity before the final catastrophe occurred in which a larger or smaller fragment of bone has broken off completely by the pull of those muscles attached to it.

Here will be described how stress can affect the hindquarter in particular, not only in avulsing portions of bone but also in producing those lesions called osteochondritis, such as of the tibial tubercle, and also how some bones or parts of bones can have secondarily an avascularity caused by a stress fracture.

The importance of a full understanding of these conditions is that the proper treatment started early may forestall the considerable morbidity that is inevitable if the patient is allowed to continue activity unabated.

Stress Avulsions of the Pelvis and Femoral Lesser Trochanter

Sporting activity plays a great part in producing stress avulsions from the pelvis which are seen from the ages of 12 to 16 in boys and girls equally. The anterior superior and inferior iliac spines are affected, as is the ischium. Invariably there has been a history of considerable activity. The patient whose radiographs are shown in Figures x.1 and x.2 was a girl of 12 who had a history of pain in the right hip which occurred during hopping and skipping. The pain was always worse in the evening and after activity. There was no sudden onset nor was there any injury. The radiograph in Figure x.1 was taken one month after the onset of symptoms and shows that part of the anterior inferior iliac spine has been avulsed but not completely separated at the top. Three months later the lesion was healing well, but it is interesting that the lower part of the avulsed fragment appears to have been absorbed rather as though it had been rendered avascular by the separation interfering with the blood supply.

A similar lesion is shown in Figures x.3 and x.4, which are the radiographs of a girl of 13 who developed pain while running. Again there was no injury and no dramatic incident.

The history of preceding symptoms is sometimes difficult to get, as with many other stress fractures, although the boy of 16 whose radiographs are shown in Figures x.5 and x.6 was quite certain that he had had seven weeks' pain, although not very severe, in the region of the anterior superior iliac spine which usually occurred during games but disappeared afterwards. He had not injured himself at all. One day running in a 100 yards race he had a sudden onset of pain which almost prevented him from running but he was able to finish the race and came second. It can be seen that he had avulsed the anterior superior iliac spine with considerable displacement but that there is callus forming already. There is no doubt that this was a long-continued process.

The radiographs should be compared to those in Figures x.7 and x.8, which are of another boy of 16 who developed sudden pain in the groin while running for a bus. Again there was no injury and the exertion was not abnormal. He was not crippled by the pain but attended hospital shortly after where the radiographs showed the avulsed anterior superior spine, which has followed exactly the same pattern as that shown in Figures x.5 and x.6. Although this boy gave no history of pain before this episode, it is very likely that this also was a stress fracture because the discomfort preceding a stress avulsion is never severe, and when the actual separation occurs pain is not crippling, as has been seen in the foregoing examples in Figures x.1 to x.6. When an injury occurs to cause a similar part to be avulsed by force, at once the symptoms are

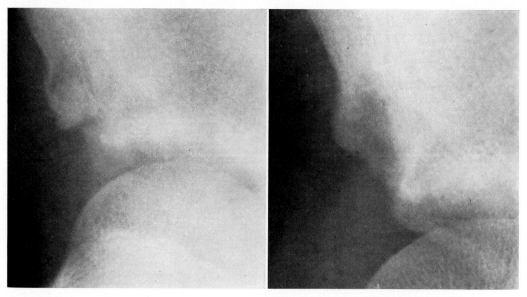

FIG. x.1   FIG. x.2

A girl aged 12 gave a history of pain in the right hip which came on during hopping and skipping. The pain was always worse in the evening and after activity. The radiograph in Figure x.1, one month after the beginning of her symptoms, shows that part of the anterior inferior iliac spine has been avulsed, but not completely. Three months later (Fig. x.2) the lesion is healing but part of the bone has been absorbed, perhaps because it was avascular.

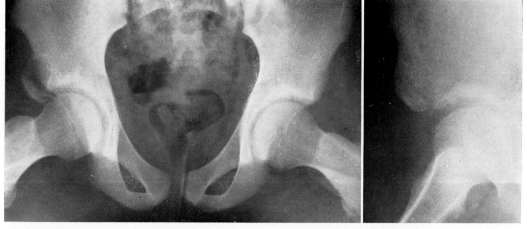

FIG. x.3   FIG. x.4

A girl of 13 sustained pain in the region of the anterior inferior iliac spine while she was running. She had had no injury. She got quite better with rest. The avulsion of the anterior inferior iliac spine is well shown, as is the unseparated apophysis of the inferior spine on the opposite side.

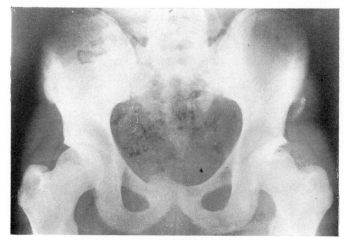
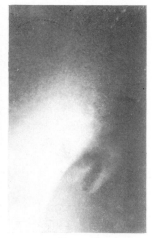

FIG. X.5   FIG. X.6

A boy of 16 had a seven weeks history of a little pain in the region of the anterior superior iliac spine which was there during games but which went off afterwards. He was certain he had not injured himself. While running in the 100 yards race he had a sudden onset of pain which almost prevented him from running but he managed to finish second. He had avulsed the anterior superior iliac spine. He was treated by rest and was allowed to start gentle training one month later.

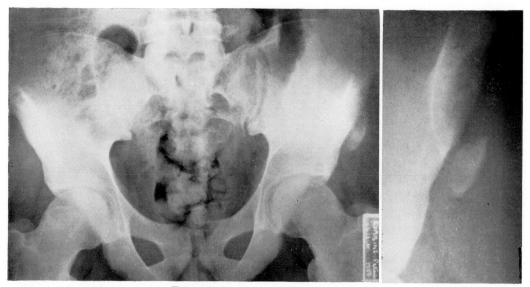

FIG. X.7   FIG. X.8

A boy of 16 developed sudden pain in the groin when running for a bus. He was found to be tender over the anterior superior iliac spine. The boy was not crippled by the pain but had to attend hospital in due course. Although there was no history of previous pain it is probable that this is a stress fracture; it did not prevent the boy from walking; a traumatic avulsion is very painful.

severe. Figures x.9 and x.10 show the radiographs of a boy of 14 who injured himself falling. He was in great pain and had to be brought to hospital, where the radiographs showed the separation of the anterior inferior iliac spine. To control the pain it was necessary to rest the boy in bed with the leg in traction.

Radiologically the lesions produced by an injury or by stress are identical in site, size and shape, and it is only the clinical history that will distinguish the two.

The ischium can have an avulsion stress injury. Figures x.11 to x.13 show the ischium of a girl of 16 who was an excellent hurdler. She always led with the left foot. Gradually she began to feel pain when taking off and finally was unable to continue her sport. When questioned she remembered that she had noticed mild twinges of a similar pain for some little while in the past. Her first radiographs show a stress fracture running into the left ischial tuberosity, which is the beginning of an avulsion of the muscular attachments to that part. Had she continued to run the whole fragment could have been avulsed.

The lesser trochanter can be avulsed. When it happens with an injury the pain at once is crippling, but when caused by continued stress the pain, although it may be bad, does not completely incapacitate the patient and gentle activity can be continued although sport has to be abandoned. Figures x.14 and x.15 shows the radiographs of a girl of 13 who was doing sport at school. During a high jump she heard a click in the left hip region and noticed some pain but this was before she had landed. On landing the pain became worse. The radiographs show the avulsion of the lesser tro-chanter and the way it was healing about one month later (Figs. x.14 and x.15).

These radiographs are very similar to those in the later stage of a similar avulsion in a boy of 13 who gradually got pain while running. He was taken off sport for some time but when he continued to have pain he was sent for advice and the radiograph in Figure x.16 shows the avulsion of the lesser trochanter.

The younger child does not get a stress avulsion near the hip since the stresses act in a different way and produce stress fractures in the inferior pubic rami. The con-ception of stress-producing lesions of different types, with different sites and with different age groups, is very important to the understanding of the implications of how various lesions can all be grouped together with one common cause, namely muscular activity.

Stress Avulsions Near the Knee

A common site for a compression stress fracture is the upper tibial shaft in an active child. Much more common, and in the same age group, is a stress avulsion of either the lower pole of the patella or of the tibial tubercle. The symptoms of these two forms of avulsion are identical and are well localised by the child to the site affected whereas the compression stress fracture of the tibia has a more vague pain and is less well localised. In all three the close association of pain at the end of activity, then during activity, but always improved by rest, is maintained.

That both the proximal and the distal end of the patellar ligament should sustain a stress avulsion is to be expected; indeed if only one end of this strap-like tendon was affected it might be more difficult to explain. The reason for the tibial tubercle being affected more often than the lower pole of the patella is explained, first, by the fact

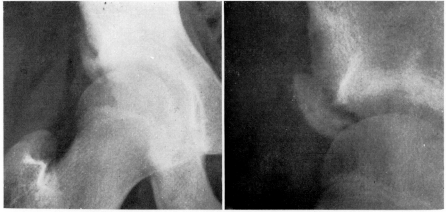

FIG. x.9   FIG. x.10

A boy of 14 fell while going up the stairs and injured his hip. He was in great pain and had to be brought to the hospital where he was found to have restriction of all right hip movements. The radiographs show a separation of the anterior inferior iliac spine. Traction was needed to relieve his pain. The opposite inferior spine showed an apophysis which had not separated. This patient shows that a traumatic avulsion is a very much more painful condition than is a stress avulsion.

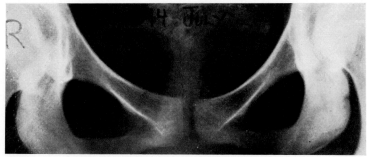

FIG. x.11

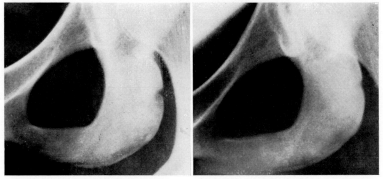

FIG. x.12   FIG. x.13

A girl of 16 was good at hurdling and led with her left foot. She began to feel pain when taking off and finally was unable to continue her sport. She had had mild twinges of a similar pain previously which caused her to take a week off from sport. The radiographs taken when she was first seen show a stress fracture in the left ischial tuberosity (Fig. x.11); this healed satisfactorily over the next few months and she was able to return to full sport. Figure x.12 was the radiograph one month later, and Figure x.13 four months after that. This stress fracture was not a complete avulsion but could well have become so without rest.

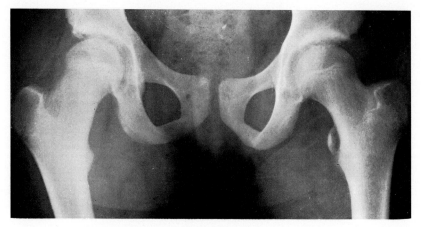

FIG. x.14

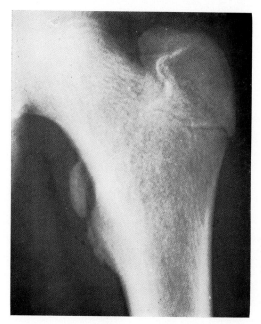

FIG. x.15

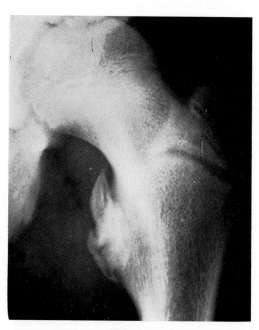

FIG. x.16

FIGS. x.14 and x.15   A girl of 13 was doing sport at school. She was doing a high jump and heard a click in the left hip region before she reached the ground and she felt the pain which became worse when she landed and she fell over. There was no pain before she felt this particular episode (Fig. x.14). Treated with rest she was much better a month later (Fig. x.15). Compare the separation of the lesser trochanter with that in Fig. x.16.

FIG. x.16   A boy aged 13 developed pain when running—and it always came on while running, despite being taken off sport for a period of time. Some two months after the onset of symptoms the lesser trochanter can be seen to have been pulled away and there is ossification around it. The appearance is very similar to that in Figure x.15.

that the lateral expansion of the quadriceps passes round the patella so that some of the muscle pull goes direct to the patellar ligament and, second, for the reason that the lateral part of the patella, particularly in children, is also subject to a stress avulsion.

Stress avulsions of the lower pole of the patella, the tibial tubercle and a lateral fragment of the patella are best described separately provided the very close association of all three is remembered. One of the few differences is a slight preponderance of boys with avulsions of the tibial tubercle but the sex incidence of avulsions of the lower pole or of a lateral fragment of the patella is the same, as are the ages of each group.

Stress Avulsions of the Lower Pole of the Patella

It is difficult to make an exact distinction between the true stress fracture of the patella and an avulsion of its lower pole, or between a stress fracture through the tibial tubercle involving the upper end of the tibia and a stress avulsion of that part. The conditions merge one into the other and, in Chapter Six on stress fractures of the patella, examples of stress avulsions of the lower pole of the patella in children were given to emphasise how the avulsions have an entirely similar symptomatology and that it is merely the size of the avulsed fragment that is different (Figs. vi.15 to vi.22). Also, in Chapter Three stress fractures of the tibial tubercle were described. These were separations of large fragments occurring in older adolescents but apart from size and age the condition was similar (Figs. iii.109 to iii.114).

The avulsion of the patellar ligament from the lower pole of the patella has been called the Sinding-Larsen Johansson syndrome, or osteochondritis of the lower pole of the patella. These names should be discarded because they are not descriptive of the condition nor do they indicate the true pathology.

Avulsions of the lower pole of the patella are often bilateral, but only if both lesions develop at the same rate will the child complain of both knees; often the more advanced lesion slows up activity to an extent that allows the opposite side to heal without symptoms. Figures x.17 to x.19 show the radiographs of the patellae of a boy aged 10 who complained of pain, swelling and giving way in the right knee for a period of six months. He particularly noticed it when he kicked. Clinically he was tender over the lower pole of the right patella. The radiograph in Figure x.17 shows the normal left patella. Figure x.18 shows an excellent example of a stress avulsion of the lower pole of the right patella. The patellar ligament has, over a few months, subjected such stress to the lower pole that it has lifted off the attachment in part and bit by bit. Figure x.19 shows the healing that had taken place with rest one month later. Figures x.20 and x.21 show the radiographs of the patellae of a boy of 13 who complained only of the left knee. The radiographs showed a stress avulsion which, had the fragment been a little bigger, could have been called a stress fracture of the lower pole of the left patella, and should be compared with the radiograph shown in Chapter Six, Figure vi.5. However, the boy, on questioning, also admitted that the right knee had been painful; the lower pole of the right patella has also been avulsed, but with trivial symptoms.

In Figures x.20 and x.21 and many subsequent radiographs the tibial tubercle has been included. This is deliberate because it is important to understand the radiological appearance of the latter and the different normal forms that are seen. The most important point is to examine the trabeculae within the tubercle for clarity and direction.

Figures x.22 to x.24 show the knees of a boy of 13 who developed pain after knocking

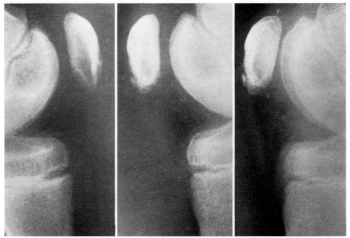

FIG. X.17   FIG. X.18   FIG. X.19

A boy of 10 complained of pain, swelling and giving way in the right knee for six months. It was worse when he kicked. He was tender over the lower pole of the right patella. He was treated by conservative methods including a plaster cylinder. He was better in one month, and Figure x.18 shows the original radiograph next to the normal left patella (Fig. x.17). Figure x.19 is one month later and shows healing.

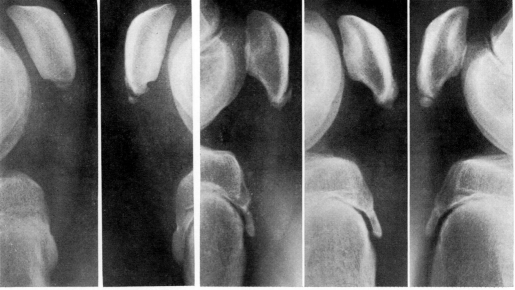

FIG. X.20   FIG. X.21   FIG. X.22   FIG. X.23   FIG. X.24

A boy of 13 had pain in his left knee with no injury but, on careful questioning, admitted also to pain in the right knee. He was tender at both lower poles. The radiograph of the left knee (Fig. x.20) shows a simple stress avulsion of the lower pole, but the right knee (Fig. x.21) has a larger lesion, though almost symptomless.

A boy of 13 hit his left knee while climbing around on some rocks and developed pain in it. This is an example of a boy who was developing a stress avulsion but had not noticed symptoms until a trivial injury brought on the pain. Figure x.22 shows the original radiograph. Two months later it was healing well (Fig. x.23) but the opposite patella showed a symptomless but similar stress fracture.

his left knee while climbing on some rocks. The injury was trivial. The lower pole of the left patella has developed a stress avulsion and two months later it has healed (Fig. x.23). At that time the right patella was radiographed, though free of symptoms, and a stress fracture across the lower pole was seen. This is not an abnormal apophysis. It had remained symptomless because the pain in the opposite knee cut down activity.

Stress Avulsion of the Tibial Tubercle

The name by which this condition is generally known is Osgood-Schlatter's disease, or osteochondritis, but, as with the lower pole of the patella, this nomenclature does not describe the condition.

The association between stress avulsion of the attachment of the patellar ligament from the lower pole of the patella by stress and its avulsion from the tibial tubercle from the same cause is closely related and is shown well in Figures x.25 to x.28, which are the radiographs of a boy of 12, who had complained a year previously of pain in his heels but these got better. No radiograph was taken at that time. A year later he attended with pain in the left knee which had come on after school sport. He was very tender in the lower pole of the left patella and the radiograph in Figure x.25 shows the avulsion of the lower pole of the patella. Notice also that the trabeculae in the left tibial tubercle appear normal. Figure x.26 shows the right knee at the same time but there is a difference between the tibial tubercles, that on the right having no trabeculation. Some five months later the lower pole of the left patella has consolidated nicely and again the left tibial tubercle is normal (Fig. x.27) but in Figure x.28 the radiograph of the right knee, again at the same time, and which had remained symptomless, shows that the tibial tubercle is beginning to develop trabeculation and has not yet united to the upper tibial epiphysis.

The direction of the trabeculae in the tibial tubercle is very important because it illustrates the continuity of force being accepted by the tibial tubercle from the tibial shaft below and the patellar ligament above. Figures x.29 to x.32 show the radiographs of the tibial tubercle of the left knee in a boy of 9 and the normal right tubercle in Figure x.33. He had noticed pain on and off and a lump in the right knee when he was first seen. Figure x.29 shows a well-advanced avulsion of the tibial tubercle. Figure x.30 shows the knee some six months later, when there is some absorption of bone on the surface but the trabeculae are beginning to run normally in the lower part of the tubercle from which it seems a portion of bone had been avulsed. Figure x.31 shows union occurring six months later, that is a year after the first radiograph, and the final state of healing 18 months after the original radiograph is shown in Figure x.32. This shows the trabeculae now running in the normal way, particularly in the lower fragment, and this can be compared to the normal right knee in Figure x.33.

Figures x.34 to x.37 show slightly different radiological pictures of stress avulsions of the tibial tubercle. They are the radiographs of a boy of 12 who had said that for some ten weeks his knees hurt at night or at the end of walking and that they were always worse after games. He was tender over both tibial tubercles. He cut down his activity and sport and was quite better in three months. The first radiographs when he was seen show that the left tubercle (Fig. x.34) was not grossly abnormal although the trabeculae were indistinct; the right tibial tubercle, however, is hazy and with a suggestion of a periosteal reaction on its anterior surface (Fig. x.35). Three months later the radiograph of the left tibial tubercle (Fig. x.36) shows periosteal new bone

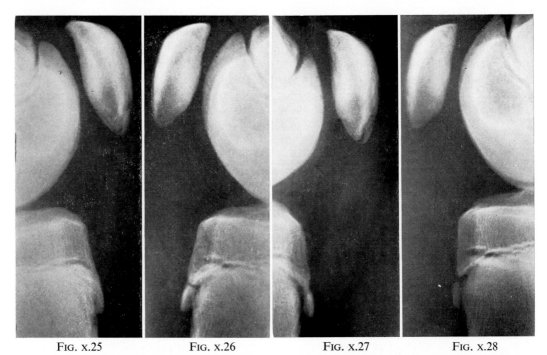

FIG. x.25   FIG. x.26   FIG. x.27   FIG. x.28

A boy of 12 complained of pain in his heels after exercise. No radiograph was taken and he got better with simple exercises but a year later he attended with pain in the left knee after long and high jumping. He was found to be very tender in the lower pole of his left patella and radiographs confirmed a stress avulsion (Fig. x.25). The left tibial tubercle is normal but that of the right knee shows no trabeculation and is small (Fig. x.26). He was free of symptoms five months later on simple restriction of activity, when further radiographs showed healing of the lower pole of the left patella (Fig. x.27) but the right tibial tubercle, although showing some trabeculation, has not become fully attached to the upper tibial epiphysis.

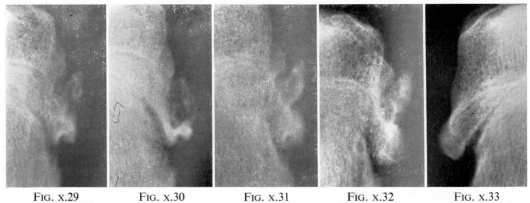

FIG. x.29   FIG. x.30   FIG. x.31   FIG. x.32   FIG. x.33

A boy of 9 noticed pain on and off in his right knee and a bump appeared. The first radiograph (Fig. x.29) shows the disrupted right tibial tubercle. The normal left tibial tubercle is shown in Figure x.33. A radiograph six months later shows some absorption taking place in the right tibial tubercle (Fig. x.30) in an effort at remodelling. A further six months later there has been consolidation of the tubercle and trabeculae are beginning to appear (Fig. x.31). Finally, after yet a further six months the healing appears to have become complete with smoothing out of the various sharp edges and trabeculae running through the tubercle in the normal way (Fig. x.32).

formation and the left trabeculae have disappeared. At this time the right tibial tubercle, in which the lesion was more advanced, shows more periosteal reaction in the radiograph (Fig. x.37), but healing has started in the lower part of the tibial tubercle and the trabeculae are beginning to show and are running in the normal direction of the line of pull of the patellar tendon.

A further example of how it is possible to recognise the avulsed tibial tubercle is shown in the radiograph in Figures x.38 to x.41. The boy in this case was 13 and had had pain in his right tibial tubercle. The left knee, in the radiograph in Figure x.38, shows the normal tibial tubercle which at first sight might have been thought to have been pulled away from its upper attachment to the upper tibial epiphysis. Instead, it has merely not yet united the apophysis to the epiphysis and, what is more, the trabeculations are normal in size and direction. However, the radiograph of the right knee, of which the boy complained, shows an entirely different formation of the tibial tubercle (Fig. x.39). The tubercle itself is fragmented and there is new bone formation around it. The proximal part also appears to have united to the epiphysis. Clinically the knee took nearly five months to heal satisfactorily at which time the good left tibial tubercle had united to the epiphysis (Fig. x.40) and the right knee by now had the trabeculations flowing in the normal direction (Fig. x.41). The characteristic bump that this condition leaves can be appreciated from the final shape of the right tibial tubercle.

It has been seen in the preceding illustrations of the boy of 13 (Figs. x.38 to x.41) that the apophysis of the tibial tubercle unites to the upper tibial epiphysis at about 13 but remains unattached to the tibia itself. At this stage of growth, when a stress avulsion occurs, peculiar patterns occur in the shape of the tibial tubercle affected (Figs. x.42 to x.45). These show the radiographs of another boy of 13 who had pain in both tibial tubercles which came on with exercise. The normal trabeculation is poor in the left tubercle (Fig. x.42) and has disappeared from the right tubercle (Fig. x.43). Healing took place in the usual way, but, when the knee was seen in radiographs two years later, as is shown in Figures x.44 and x.45, both tibial tubercles had healed but leaving an extension upwards in one and a large beak in the other; the normal direction of the trabeculae is obvious. At this time the tubercles are uniting to the upper tibial shaft.

When, with normal activity, excess stress is applied to the region of the tibial tubercle after it has united to the tibial metaphysis, a different pattern of reaction is apparent. Figures x.46 and x.47 are the radiographs of a man of 19 who had had pain in the right tibial tubercle for two years preceded by pain in the left. The peculiar indentation which is seen below the tibial tubercle on each side is a stress fracture which has, as it were, aborted and has not become complete. Had it become complete the condition shown in the adjacent Figures of x.48 and x.49 would have occurred. Both the latter radiographs of complete stress fractures of the tibial tubercle are also shown in Chapter Three, Figures III.109 to III.114, where they are described in full. The radiograph in Figure x.48 demonstrates that the stress fracture at the age of 16, when there is solid union of the tibial tubercle to both epiphysis and metaphysis, allows the avulsion of a whole piece of both tubercle and upper tibial epiphysis to occur. Figure x.49, the radiograph of a girl of 14, shows that if the tubercle has not fully united to the tibial metaphysis it will sustain a stress fracture at the junction of the tubercle to the epiphysis.

O

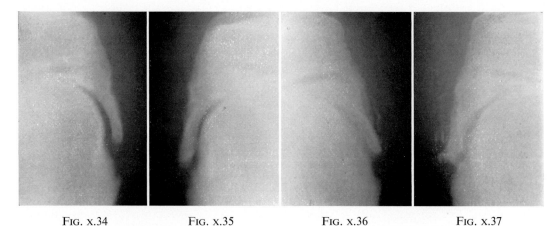

FIG. X.34   FIG. X.35   FIG. X.36   FIG. X.37

A boy of 12 said that his knees had hurt at night or at the end of walking for some 10 weeks and that the pain was always worse after games. He was tender over both tibial tubercles. He was advised to cut down his exercise. The first radiographs show an almost normal left tibial tubercle but the trabeculae are indistinct (Fig. x.34) when he was first seen. The right tibial tubercle has a more advanced stress avulsion and there is some periosteal new bone formation anteriorly. The trabeculae have disappeared (Fig. x.35). Three months later the lesion of the left tibial tubercle is much more obvious (Fig. x.36), whereas the right tubercle is healing with clear evidence of trabeculae running in the line of the pull of the patellar tendon (Fig. x.37).

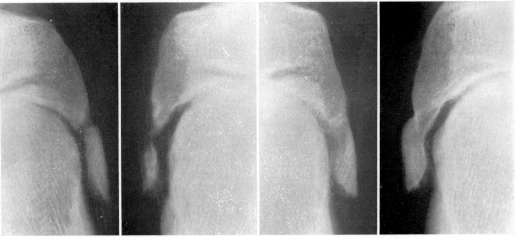

FIG. X.38   FIG. X.39   FIG. X.40   FIG. X.41

A boy of 13 had had a slight knock on the right tibial tubercle, and thereafter had pain. It was a trivial injury. The apophysis for the left, or unaffected, tibial tubercle (Fig. x.38) is clear-cut with good trabeculae but is not yet united to the epiphysis, whereas the right tibial tubercle has united the proximal part, is fragmented and has lost the trabeculae (Fig. x.39). Five months later the left tubercle was joined to the epiphysis in the normal way (Fig. x.40) but the right, or affected, tubercle shows considerable deformity, but has healed as is shown by the reformation of the normal trabecular pattern (Fig. x.41).

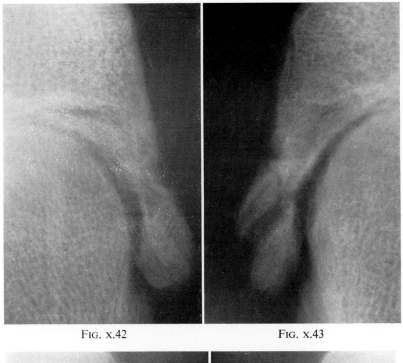

FIG. x.42   FIG. x.43

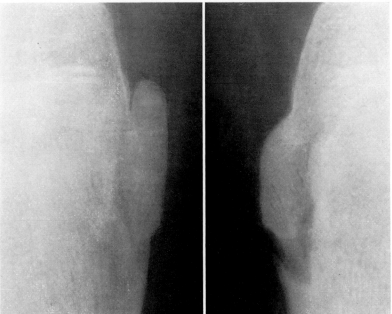

FIG. x.44   FIG. x.45

A boy of 13 had pain in both tibial tubercles made worse by exercise. The initial radiographs demonstrate the early loss of the trabeculae, less on the left (Fig. x.42) than on the right (Fig. x.43). Two years later the difference in the manner of healing of each tubercle is shown in the radiographs in Figures x.44 and x.45. The trabeculae are normal in direction and the tubercles are uniting to the tibial metaphysis.

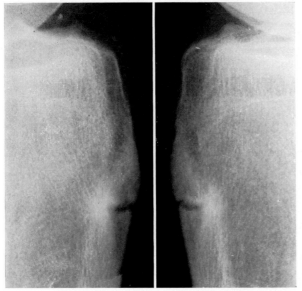

FIG. X.46   FIG. X.47

FIGS. X.46 and X.47   A man aged 19 had had pain in the right knee for two years, and before that in the left. Recently more pain in the right knee caused him to attend hospital because he thought he had strained it. He was found to be very tender on both tibia just below the joint line and on each side of the insertion of the patella ligament. The peculiar radiological appearance is of a stress fracture that had never become complete. This appearance is very like that in the ischium shown in Figures X.11 and X.12.

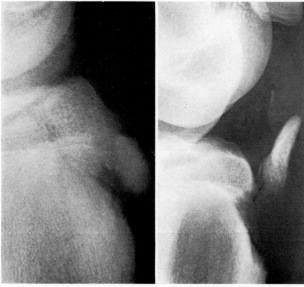

FIG. X.48   FIG. X.49

FIG. X.48   The boy in this radiograph has been described in Chapter Three, Figures III.109 and III.111. He had a typical history of a stress fracture for some two years with pain in the region of the tibial tubercle but always after energetic activity. One day, running over flat ground, with no injury, he felt pain in the knee and fell to the ground. He had had a stress fracture which had become complete and because the tubercle was uniting to the metaphysis part of the epiphysis was avulsed as well.

FIG. X.49   A schoolgirl of 14 of championship status had noticed pain just below the left knee throughout the summer while running and jumping. She has been described in Chapter Three, Figures III.112 and III.114. Suddenly she felt a pain in the knee and collapsed. She had avulsed her tibial tubercle although it was already well united to the upper tibial epiphysis. A small amount of new bone formation is visible on the posterior surface of the tubercle indicating that the stress lesion was not a sudden traumatic avulsion.

The Bipartite Patella

It has been shown in Chapter Six that there is a stress fracture of the lateral margin of the patella. The child with a bipartite patella can have the smaller fragment partially avulsed by stress and this gives rise to symptoms. One such case has already been described in an older boy in Figures vi.9 and vi.10 in Chapter Six. The bipartite fragment may be in the proximal and lateral quadrant of the patella or in the distal and lateral part, but the symptoms are the same in each case and to those of stress fractures in general. There is, however, a difference because the avulsed fragment having articular cartilage on it may develop chondromalacia and the symptoms thereof.

It is possible that some of the bipartite fragments are in fact ununited stress avulsions from an early age and before the patella has become partly or completely ossified. If a small part is avulsed, as in the stress fracture in the adult, it may remain ununited and separate. Figures x.50 to x.53 show the development of a bipartite patella after a 'twist' which could hardly have applied the force necessary to cause a traumatic disruption. In this case the separation of the smaller fragment was quite marked and greatly in excess of the 'normal' bipartite fragment. Excision was necessary. The more usual findings of a painful bipartite patella are shown in Figures x.54 and x.55, being the radiographs of the knees of a boy of 12. In Figure x.54 the unilateral bipartite patella is seen to be in the proximal and lateral part of the patella. It caused considerable symptoms, and the boy got pain severe enough to cause him to limp, especially with any increase of activity. The right knee was normal. The lateral radiograph of the left knee in Figure x.55 suggests that the smaller fragment had moved in relation to the larger. Conservative treatment failed and the small fragment was excised with complete recovery.

Figures x.56 and x.57 show the radiographs of the knees of a girl of 12. She had the other kind of bipartite patella, bilateral, and in the distal and lateral part of the patella. Again conservative treatment failed to produce any improvement in the pain and 'giving way' of the knees, which even caused her to fall to the ground, and first one and then the other fragment was excised with complete cure. Figure x.56 shows the anteroposterior radiograph of both knees after the fragment had been excised from the left knee, and Figure x.57 shows the tangential views, again after excision of the left fragment; in this radiograph the gap whence the small fragment was excised looks as though the fragment did not actually involve the joint surface, but that this is an illusion is apparent when the antero-posterior radiograph (Fig. x.56) is studied. Always at operation it is found that the fragment is covered by a small area of joint cartilage. The fragment in the tangential view of the right patella also gives the appearance of having moved out of its normal position in regard to the rest of the patella.

Although the bipartite patella may on many occasions give rise to no symptoms, should there be good reason to believe that the fragment is causing disability then it should be excised because the result is always extremely good, followed by a rapid return to function.

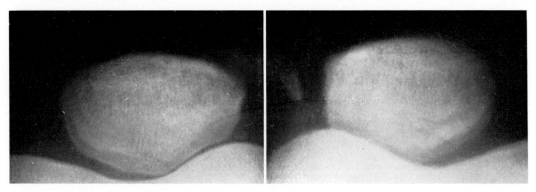

FIG. x.50   FIG. x.51

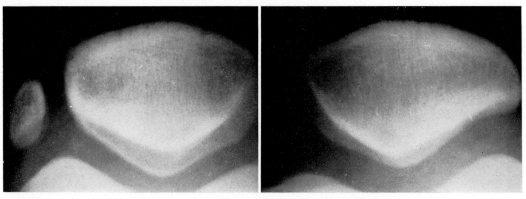

FIG. x.52   FIG. x.53

This interesting boy at the age of 11 was said to have twisted the right knee playing football. He had slight pain on full extension with tenderness over and below the patella. The radiograph was normal and a tangential view also showed no abnormality (Fig. x.50). He got better quickly but returned two months later with tenderness over the lower and lateral border of the patella and flexion of the knee was reduced by pain. A month later the radiograph, again a tangential view, showed a very small piece of bone on the lateral aspect (Fig. x.51); the knee then got better. For a further 18 months there was little trouble but then he complained that the knee used to 'stick' and he could feel a little lump on the outer side of the kneecap. The lump appeared to the patient to come, or to go, with more, or less, movement of the knee. The ossicle in the radiograph (Fig. x.52) had grown with the patella; the ossicle was then excised at operation. Macroscopically the join was fibro-cartilaginous tissue. A few months later the boy reported that for the first time his knee did not trouble him at all. A year later the radiograph was normal (Fig. x.53).

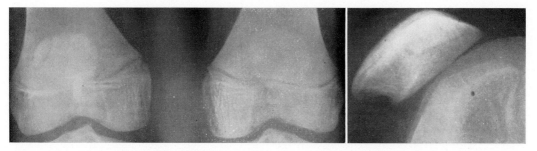

FIG. x.54   FIG. x.55

A boy of 12 had pain in the right knee which caused him to limp when he was being active. He was found to be very tender in the lateral part of the right patella. Two months later that part was removed and follow-up a year later showed the boy to be entirely better. The radiograph in Figure x.54 shows that he had a unilateral bipartite patella in the proximal and lateral part. The lateral view in Figure x.55 suggests that the small fragment has moved from its proper bed.

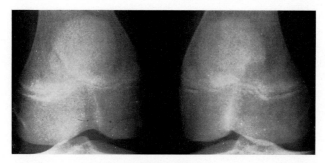

FIG. x.56

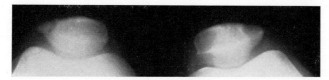

FIG. x.57

FIGS. x.56 and x.57   A girl of 12 complained of both knees giving way, the left being worse than the right, and it even let her fall to the floor. She had much pain around the kneecap. She said that when she knelt she felt as if she was kneeling on broken glass. Conservative treatment failed and six months later the left bipartite fragment was removed which made her knee so much better that she demanded to have the other side done. The deep surface of the patella showed slight chondromalacia. Figure x.56 shows the site of the bipartite fragments, the left fragment having already been excised. The tangential radiograph in Figure x.57 suggests that the fragment on the left did not involve the joint surface but this was not found to be so at operation, nor is it suggested in the anteroposterior radiograph in Figure x.56.

Avascular Necrosis

To obtain conclusive evidence that avascular necrosis of a bone in childhood is directly caused by a stress fracture is difficult but on clinical grounds there is ample evidence to suggest that some, if not all, cases are caused in this way.

Perthes' disease of the hip may be unilateral or bilateral but from the moment that the child has first complained of a little pain in the hip the progress is remorseless. It is possible that treatment may alter to some extent the shape and amount of avascularity of the femoral head but, in the main, the condition has been predestined from the earliest stage and probably before the child has ever started to complain. One of the very few conditions which can fit the causation of most cases of Perthes' disease is that there has been a compression stress fracture actually within the femoral head. The extent of such a stress fracture would be variable and would cause more or less avascularity accordingly.

It has been shown that the stress fracture of the head of the femur is a cause of the idiopathic avascular necrosis that is seen in the adult. It has also been shown that a stress fracture of the pubic ramus is quite common in the older patient. Also, stress fractures of the pubic ramus are seen in the child. However, the child at the age when a pubic stress fracture occurs is also susceptible to Perthes' disease, again as the older patient is to stress fractures of the femoral head with avascular necrosis.

Children do not get stress fractures of the neck of the femur although it is seen at all ages after the upper epiphysial plate of the femur has closed. Before the growth plate has closed Perthes' disease is seen in the younger child and the chronic slipping of the upper femoral epiphysis in the older child. The latter is a stress fracture through the metaphysial aspect of the growth plate of which condition the history of pain with activity and gradually getting worse is typical.

In Perthes' disease, as in all other examples of juvenile idiopathic osteochondritis, once the bone has become dense the stress fracture is no longer visible and indeed has probably already been absorbed, because the healing is very rapid in the child. It does, however, leave behind it the dead or partly dead femoral head. It is not difficult to assume that this can occur even with a very small amount of compression of the cancellous bone in the femoral head: it is not necessary to block the arteries, simple venous occlusion will cause avascularity.

The child who has a stress fracture of the upper tibia can have a very slight haze of callus showing in the radiograph, if indeed there is anything to be seen, when he first attends. With this stress fracture the child complains of a slight ache in the knee or pain after exercise. The symptoms are not severe: signs can be very slight. The same symptoms occur in the first instance with Perthes' disease but once the blood supply to the femoral head has been affected further symptoms will accrue. The child admitted for observation of the hip because of a limp and some pain is often found to have a stress fracture of the pubic ramus. The symptoms of a stress fracture in this part mimic the early stage of Perthes' disease.

As yet no clear and indisputable radiological confirmation has been found to confirm this cause of Perthes' disease. The reasons for this are either that a stress fracture of the femoral head in the child is not a cause of Perthes' disease of the hip or that, by the time symptoms appear and the hip is radiographed, the haze of internal callus is too faint to be seen.

If it could be shown that other forms of a similar condition, such as Köhler's disease of the navicular bone, Freiberg's infraction of a metatarsal head or Sever's disease of the calcaneal epiphysis were the result of a stress fracture, then the support for the same aetiology in Perthes' disease would be very great. Such evidence, in fact, exists.

Stress fractures of the navicular bone in adults have been described in Chapter Eight. It would be surprising if there was not a similar condition in childhood. Radiological confirmation has to be very early and preferably before continued walking causes the condition to advance so far that the initial stress fracture cannot be seen. Figures x.58 and x.59 show the radiographs of the right foot in a boy of 6. He had chorea and had been admitted to hospital and the condition in the right navicular bone was found incidentally. Comparing the navicular bones, that on the right has a quite obvious compression stress fracture within the bone which is slightly flattened with less depth than that on the left. The part of the right navicular bone proximal to the fracture does not have a different density from that of the opposite bone. A short while later complete resolution had occurred and the bone had healed with no further deformity (Fig. x.59).

Another form which this condition can take is shown in Figure x.60. Here the radiograph of the navicular bone of a boy aged 6 has become avascular but with a fracture line passing distally through the centre of the bone. It is exactly in this direction that the stress fractures lie in the adult, as shown in Figures viii.19 to viii.22.

Freiberg's infraction of the metatarsal head has been seen to be the result of a stress fracture at the base of the metatarsal head and was discussed in Chapter Eight, Figures viii.47 and viii.48. The condition is the late result of avascular necrosis of the femoral head after a compression stress fracture. Such stress fractures show only a very slight haze of internal callus but the latter is well demonstrated in the metatarsal necks of a child with march fractures in Chapter Eight, Figures viii.47 and viii.48. In the radiographs in Figures x.61 to x.63, which are of a girl of 8, the haze of internal callus can be seen in the third metatarsal head. The second radiograph (Fig. x.62), only three weeks later, shows the stress fracture better with a fracture line actually across the dense area. Figure x.63 shows the final outcome with deformity obvious though slight.

Sever's disease of the apophysis of the calcaneum has been described in Chapter Eight, Figures viii.11 to viii.18, when it was shown to be a stress fracture of the apophysis. The gradual course of the symptoms and radiological signs of this condition from the beginning to complete recovery follows in many respects—except position— that of the navicular bone with Köhler's disease. Another example is shown in Figures x.64 to x.71. The increase in density of the apophysis is occasioned by the callus that builds up within the apophysis; with healing, the lesion resolves and the apophysis becomes normal. The symptoms are typical of a stress fracture. The apophysis is being compressed by the same forces that cause a compression stress fracture of the calcaneum.

From the foregoing it is apparent that a very slight compression of a child's bone can occur; and that when it occurs in certain places it has been shown to cause avascular necrosis. As a clinical corollary it is to be expected that avascular necrosis in the hip might have the same cause.

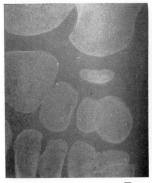
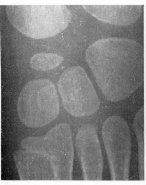
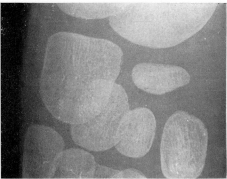

FIG. x.58

FIG. x.59

FIGS. x.58 and x.59   A boy of 6 was admitted to hospital for investigation of chorea and was found incidentally to have Köhler's disease of the right navicular bone (Fig. x.58). The radiographs show that the right navicular bone is only very slightly smaller than the left, but that there is a definite haze of internal callus within it. Only the distal part of the bone has been affected, and the proximal part has the same density as the opposite navicular bone. The whole of the right navicular bone has not gone avascular after the stress fracture probably because the child was not walking on it. Figure x.59 shows the complete recovery and restoration of shape that occurred.

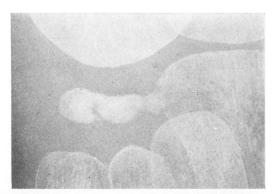

FIG. x.60   A typical example of Köhler's disease of the left navicular bone in a boy of 6. Here the whole of the bone has been compressed after going avascular but there is a fracture line down the centre of the bone, which follows the same direction as the stress fracture of this bone seen in the adult.

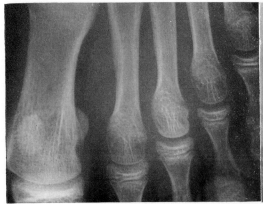
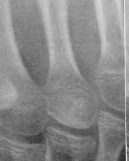
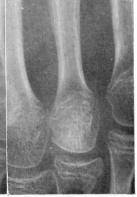

FIG. x.61

FIG. x.62

FIG. x.63

A girl of 8 was admitted with pain in the foot ascribed to 'rheumatism'. Examination revealed a compression stress fracture of the third metatarsal head. In Figure x.61 little more than increased density can be seen. In Figure x.62 three weeks later the fracture is evident, and Figure x.63 shows the typical—but slight—deformity which developed despite the avoidance of weight-bearing.

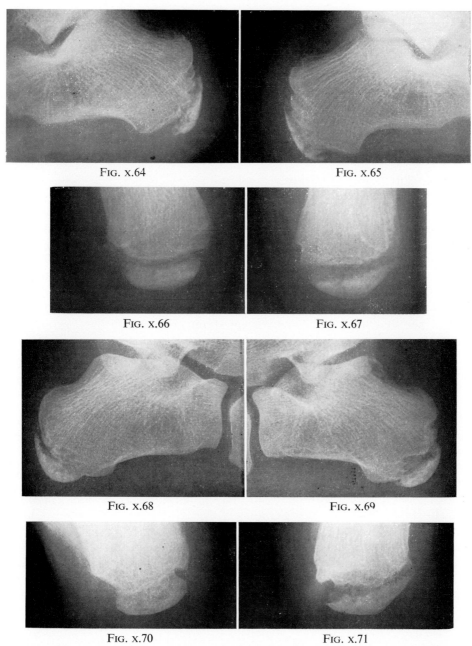

FIG. X.64   FIG. X.65

FIG. X.66   FIG. X.67

FIG. X.68   FIG. X.69

FIG. X.70   FIG. X.71

A boy of 11 had had intermittent pain in his heels for about a year. For about one month before he was first seen he had suffered more pain in the right heel than in the left. The radiographs show that the apophysis of the right calcaneus in the lateral view (Fig. x.64) is slightly dense, but the left apophysis is more dense, with fragmentation. The tangential views show that the left apophysis (Fig. x.67) has a well-developed compression stress fracture which is healing, but the right apophysis (Fig. x.66) has the much slighter and less well-marked internal callus of a developing compression stress fracture. Five weeks later, after using thick sorbo rubber heel pads, his symptoms had stopped and the radiographs show the healing of the left apophysis (Figs. x.69 and x.71) and healing progressing in the right apophysis (Figs. x.68 and x.70). Compare these radiographs to those in Figures VIII.11 to VIII.18, page 153.

CHAPTER ELEVEN

COMPARATIVE STRESS FRACTURES

Stress Fractures in Horses

There is a condition in horses known as splint disease, which is lameness with swelling of the foreleg of the horse—a part comparable to the human shin and consisting of the cannon bone, which is the third metacarpal bone, with two splint bones, one on each side, being respectively the vestigial remnants of the second and fourth metacarpal bones (Fig. XI.1). There is an interosseous ligament between each splint bone and the cannon bone. At about the age of 7 years the splint bones become ossified to the cannon or third metacarpal bone. Proximally they take part in the carpometacarpal joint and it is thought that they can take weight which is passed through the interosseous ligament to the third metacarpal bone. At first the condition was thought to be a traumatic inflammation of the medial splint bone, hence the name. With the advent of radiography the condition also became known as metacarpal periostitis.

A yearling or a two-year-old in training will suddenly 'buck', that is go lame on one foreleg, and there is even evidence to believe that there are prodromal symptoms because trainers will speak of a horse as being about to buck.

After going lame a swelling appears on the medial side of the cannon bone. It is this bone that resembles the human shin in being long, thin and subcutaneous. The swelling that occurs is easily visible (Figs. XI.2 and XI.3) and, as is the case in the athlete, it is always hard to the examining finger. Gradually, if the horse is correctly treated, the swelling begins to get less although in part it may remain permanently. Training can be continued after a very variable period of time with no ill effects. However, if training does start again too soon then it is found that the horse 'bucks its shin' again.

The radiographic findings—being consistent over a considerable number of horses—indicate that this condition is a stress fracture comparable to 'shin soreness' in an athlete. It is interesting that the condition in the athlete and the horse both occur at relatively the same age, that is when both horse and athlete are reaching skeletal maturity. It is also interesting that the name of the condition to sportsmen is extremely similar—shin soreness or sore shins being so similar that it seemed that there must be a connection, at any rate in the sportsman's mind. The first horse to be seen with this condition (Figs. XI.2 and XI.3) was typical of the condition. She was a two-year-old thoroughbred who went lame while training. There was no evidence of injury. She was confined to her stall on soft litter and she improved slowly.

The radiographs shown in Figures XI.4 and XI.5 show that the stress fracture can be seen running upwards and laterally in the lower-most third of the cannon—or third metacarpal—bone of the left foreleg with good callus surrounding it.

The horse was treated in the same way as is an athlete, by rest. It is difficult to achieve this satisfactorily in a horse which has to stay on its feet, but, provided it is kept in a

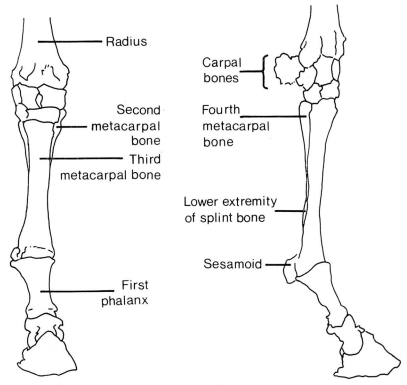

FIG. XI.1

The anatomy of the foreleg of the horse.

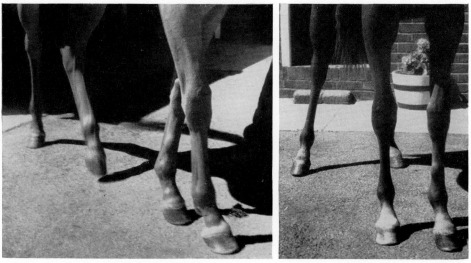

FIG. XI.2   FIG. XI.3

Clinical photographs of a two-year-old horse who developed splint disease of the left foreleg. The swelling on the shin is shown very well. There was no history of injury and the only activities had been training on reasonably firm ground with no untoward features in the landscape to account for a hidden injury.

stall with a firm but soft litter, it is able to take the weight more effectively on the other three members. Unlike the dog, the horse cannot manage on three legs holding the fourth aloft.

The horse cannot complain and therefore rest should be sufficiently long to allow complete healing of the fracture, which can best be assessed by serial radiography. However, horses become frisky and restive and are not easy to radiograph in such a way as to show clear bone detail.

In just the same way that it is difficult to know when a horse has slight pain as it cannot complain before actually going lame, so it is difficult for the trainer to know when the horse is free of symptoms because the swelling does not necessarily disappear. The horse in Figures XI.2 to XI.5 had less swelling after a year but had returned to racing and had been placed on several occasions.

The radiographs shown in Figures XI.4 and XI.5 are above two radiographs of athletes (Figs. XI.6 and XI.7), both of whose stress fractures have been dealt with earlier in Chapter Three, Figures III.32 to III.37 and III.43. The fracture line in Figures XI.4 and XI.6 can be seen going upwards and towards the centre of the bone very clearly. The callus on the outer side of the fracture line is also shown in the antero-posterior view in Figure XI.4, and early callus is forming around the fracture line in Figure XI.6. Figure XI.5 is a lateral view of the third metacarpal, or cannon bone, and the callus appears in this to have involved the medial splint which lies close to the cannon bone. The splint bone is firmly bound down to the cannon bone by an inter-osseous ligament and therefore callus in this area must displace the splint bone. How-ever, the callus formation on the cannon bone is very similar to that in Figure XI.7. It was this radiographic finding that caused the condition to be considered periostitis.

Another two-year-old thoroughbred had a history of bucked shins six weeks before the radiograph shown in Figure XI.8 was taken. Figure XI.9 is an enlarged view of the radiograph, showing in greater detail the periosteal new bone formation. Next to this figure is the radiograph of the tibia of an athlete with shin soreness (Fig. XI.10). The periosteal new bone formation of both horse and athlete is very much alike. Figure XI.11 shows a later stage in the progress of the same stress fracture in the athlete whose tibia is shown in Figure XI.10; the fracture line can now be seen running upwards and towards the centre of the bone, and callus has increased. Adjacent is Figure XI.12, that of another two-year-old horse. Here again the callus is abundant and, although radiographic quality is not very good, the fracture line can be seen running upwards and towards the centre of the bone. As in the athlete with this condition only one cortex has been involved.

Figure XI.13 shows the radiograph of the cannon bone of a yearling with rather a long area of new bone formation. Whether in fact this could be related to the more longitudinal fractures seen occasionally in the athlete is doubtful, but this particular horse, because of the apparent involvement of the splint bone and its suspensory ligaments which lie between it and the third metacarpal bone, was operated upon and the callus removed. The radiograph after operation (Fig. XI.14) shows where the bone has been removed but also confirms that there is a fracture line which runs up and inwards through the medial cortex. The medial cortex in this area is thickened; these radiographs should be compared to those of an athlete (Figs. XI.15 and XI.16) in whom the callus in one view appeared to involve and press upon the fibula. Tomographs showed that the lesion was entirely confined to the cortex of the tibia on its postero-

FIGS. XI.4 and XI.5 Radiographs of the right foreleg of the horse shown in Figures XI.2 and XI.3. The metacarpal—or cannon—bone has a fracture line running upwards and inwards (Fig. XI.4) exactly as in the shin soreness type of stress fracture in the athlete, an example of which is given for comparison in Figure XI.6 below. The lateral view (Fig. XI.5) shows how the medial splint bone, which is a remnant of the second metacarpal bone, appears to be involved in the callus. However, since the anteroposterior view shows a great deal more callus, it is merely that the splint bone has been pushed away from the cannon bone by enlarging callus.

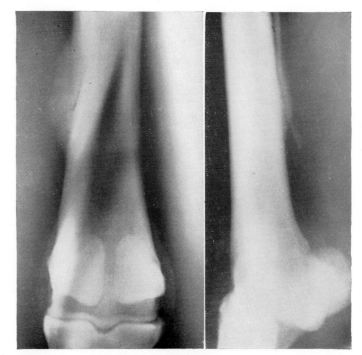

FIG. XI.4   FIG. XI.5

FIG. XI.6 An athlete described earlier in this book (Figs. III.32 to III.37) developed shin soreness. The fracture is very similar to that shown in Figure XI.4.

FIG. XI.7. Another athlete described earlier in Chapter Three (Fig. III.43) had a radiograph showing callus around a stress fracture which is very like that shown in Figure XI.5.

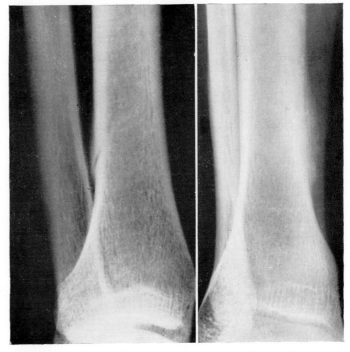

FIG. XI.6   FIG. XI.7

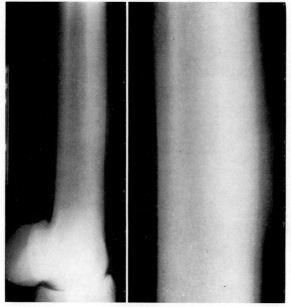

FIG. XI.8   FIG. XI.9   FIG. XI.10

The radiograph of the left foreleg of a two-year-old thoroughbred who had a history of bucked shins of six weeks (Fig. XI.8). The radiographs show a small area of periosteal new bone formation which is more clearly shown in the enlarged view in Figure XI.9.

This radiograph shows the periosteal new bone formation in an athlete who had sore shins. This was the earliest change to be found in this particular patient and it compares very well to that seen in the radiographs of the horse shown in Figures XI.8 and XI.9.

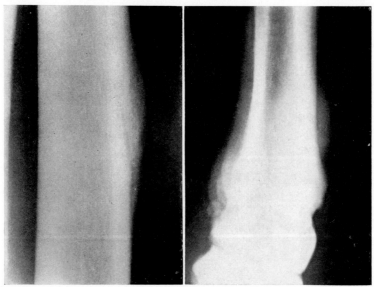

FIG. XI.11   FIG. XI.12

Figure XI.11 is a radiograph taken later in the development of the stress fracture in the patient in the last radiograph (Fig. XI.10) which is to be compared to Figure XI.12, the radiograph of a two-year-old thoroughbred in which the fracture can be seen running upwards and inwards.

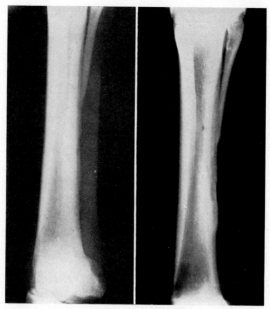

FIG. XI.13   FIG. XI.14

The radiograph of the third metacarpal bone of a yearling which was thought to have periostitis and which appeared to involve the medial splint—or second metacarpal—bone (Fig. XI.13). As it was considered that the suspensory ligament (an important structure in the shin of the horse) was being involved, the callus was excised and the radiograph after operation is shown in Figure XI.14. Here the fracture line can still be seen running upwards and inwards. However, the callus and thickening of the cortex is well shown in Figure XI.13 and can be compared to the figures below, the radiographs of the tibia of an athlete.

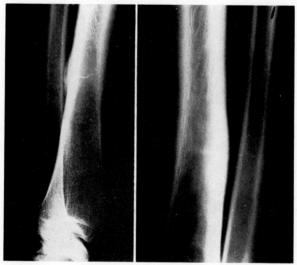

FIG. XI.15   FIG. XI.16

These radiographs show the stress fracture in an 18-year-old medical student. In an oblique view (Fig. X.15) the callus on the tibia and the thickening of its cortex does not show a fracture very clearly, and appears to be involving the fibula and even to have eroded it slightly. This is purely a radiological illusion, confirmed as such by the tomographs (Fig. XI.16), which showed that the callus was entirely from the tibia and had not even broken the periosteum.

P

lateral aspect (Fig. XI.16). The involvement of the splint bone (Fig. XI.13) was as illusory as it was of the fibula of the athlete.

Other radiographs of the appearance of a stress fracture of the cannon bone in horses are shown in Figures XI.17 to XI.19. In the first radiograph the fracture is higher than is usual but still runs upwards and inwards. At this level in the athlete it is usual to find the fracture running downwards and towards the centre of the bone. Figure XI.18 is typical of splint disease with just a small area of compact subperiosteal new bone formation, such as is so frequently seen in athletes. Figure XI.19 is interesting in that the radiograph was taken very late and the callus is not only mature but absorbing, which has caused the slight irregularities in its surface.

Figures XI.20 to XI.22 are radiographs of the tibiae in athletes with shin soreness, all of whom have been described in Chapter Three (Figs. III.42, III.53 and III.55).

There is another condition in horses known as a fissure fracture of the cannon bone, and such a one is shown in Figures XI.23 and XI.24. This occurred in a thoroughbred gelding aged 11 years. He had run quite well in a race but some hours later when being taken out of his stable to be taken home he put half the forefoot on a concrete path. When he took his weight the forefoot slipped off the side of the concrete and went down some 4 to 6 inches with considerable force. He immediately became lame. This is a traumatic fracture, not a stress fracture, and must not be confused with the usual stress fracture. The same condition can occur in the human, and the radiographs of a girl who had a similar sort of injury are shown in Figures XI.25 and XI.26. The medial malleolus has been sheared off in very much the same way as has the lower part of the cannon bone. The girl also has a fracture of the lateral malleolus.

The evidence for most, if not all, of splint disease being a stress fracture is very convincing and, with the further use of radiography in training stables, treatment by the usual method of rest will become far more effective because the young horse will be kept from training until there is radiological union which is satisfactory. Then the training should be slow and graduated as for the athlete.

'Splints', or splint disease, has been thought to be a different disease from 'sore shins' but the two lesions are stress fractures occurring in different parts of the cannon bone.

Without a full understanding of the condition, proper treatment will not be based on the true pathology and a potential champion racehorse might be deprived of success because of a too hurried return to training, or by having outmoded treatment, which, giving insufficient rest, cause much hardship and distress—as it may also do in the ill-treated athlete.

Stress Fractures in the Greyhound

The navicular (tarsal scaphoid) bone in the greyhound sustains a stress fracture, and the great interest in this particular lesion is that it almost always occurs in the right navicular bone. The stress fracture that occurs is not unlike that seen in the human navicular bone (Chapter Eight, Figs. VIII.19 to VIII.22) but because it becomes complete there is usually some displacement of part of the bone.

The greyhound races anticlockwise on the track and, as can be seen from Figures XI.27 to XI.29, the thrust on the right hindleg is very considerable when the dogs are travelling at speed. Greyhounds can achieve speeds around 30 miles an hour or more.

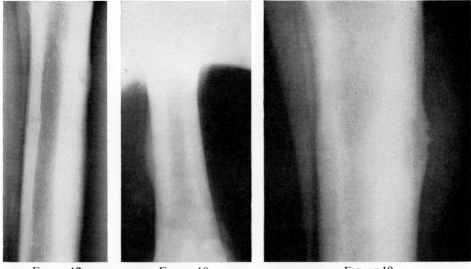

FIG. XI.17   FIG. XI.18   FIG. XI.19

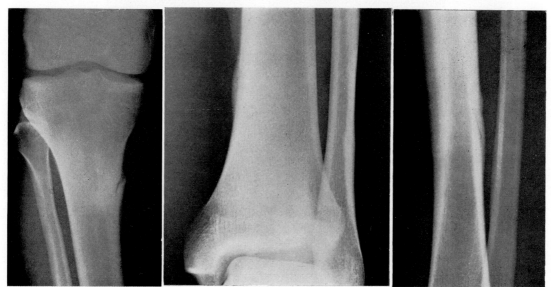

FIG. XI.20   FIG. XI.21   FIG. XI.22

The six radiographs shown here are for comparison and especially to show that both horse and man can have a very variable radiological presentation of a stress fracture even in one particular group. The radiographs at the top are all of yearlings or two-year-olds and those at the bottom from young athletes. Figure XI.17 shows an incomplete stress fracture which only goes through the anteromedial cortex of the cannon bone. It is very similar to that seen in the athlete with shin soreness but the fracture runs upwards and not downwards, as it does in the athlete, when it is in the uppermost third of the tibia. A radiograph of the tibia of an athlete with shin soreness is shown in Figure XI.20 for comparison. Figure XI.18 shows periosteal callus, again very typical of the milder form of shin soreness, and is above Figure XI.21, again the radiograph of a young athlete with shin soreness. A late stage of the same condition in another horse is shown in Figure XI.19. Here the callus is being eroded and absorbed because the stress fracture has united. Compare this with Figure XI.22, which is the radiograph of a healing stress fracture of the tibia in an athlete.

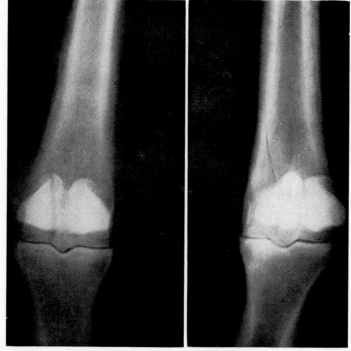

FIG. XI.23   FIG. XI.24

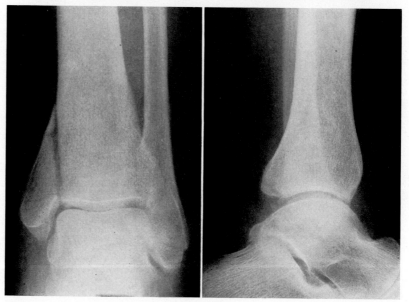

FIG. XI.25   FIG. XI.26

These radiographs are not of stress fractures. Figures XI.23 and XI.24 are two radiographs of an 11-year-old horse, a thoroughbred gelding with a 'fissure' fracture caused by the hoof slipping off a concrete pathway. The third metacarpal, or cannon, bone has had a fracture of its lowest third involving the metacarpophalangeal joint. Figures XI.25 and XI.26 are radiographs of a similar injury in a young adult. The fissure fracture in the horse must not be confused with a stress fracture.

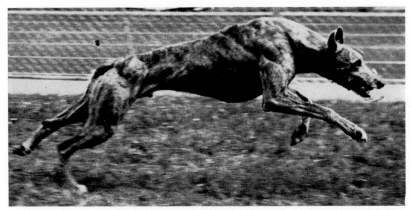

FIG. XI.27

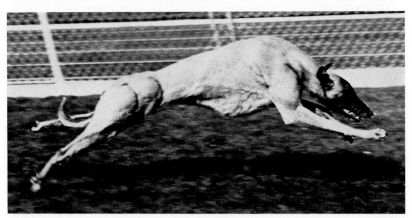

FIG. XI.28

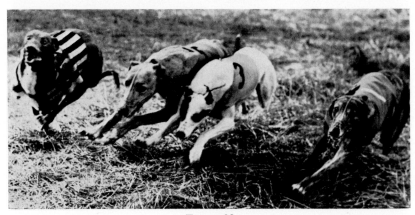

FIG. XI.29

Greyhounds racing at speed. These illustrations show the great effort used by the greyhounds and the extremely large range of movement that there is in the ankle. Figure XI.29 shows how the greyhounds corner. Notice particularly how the dog on the left of the picture is cornering with the left hindleg tucked well underneath the body thus using gravity to assist in the turn to the left.

The extra force required to change direction continually to the left, in going round the racing track anticlockwise, also gives an additional burden to the right hindleg.

Examination of the navicular bones from trained greyhounds clearly indicates which side is which, quite apart from the anatomical difference, because the right navicular bone has, in the fresh specimen, reddish staining of the whole bone (Figs. XI.30 and XI.31). This indicates that there has been considerable bruising within the bone during the lifetime of the dog. Such bruising is also seen in the left navicular bone but to a much lesser extent. In navicular bones which have been removed after stress fractures this heavy bruising is always to be seen.

The trained observer can often identify a particular moment in the race when the greyhound gets, or is likely to get, this fracture. Figure XI.29 shows greyhounds cornering at speed. The greyhound on the left has the left hindleg tucked well underneath the body, which is leaning over to the left. Gravity will now assist the cornering to the left in the same way that it does for the motor-cyclist. If, through a failure of technique, the greyhound has to corner on the right hindleg, the additional thrust necessary may, on occasion, be the moment when the stress fracture becomes complete. Figure XI.30 shows a dried specimen of a greyhound's navicular bone with an undisplaced stress fracture. Adjacent, in Figure XI.31, is a fresh specimen showing the heavy bruising so characteristic of the right navicular bone, but with no macroscopical fracture to be seen.

Figures XI.32 and XI.33 show radiographs of a stress fracture of the navicular bone of the greyhound.

Treatment is interesting because, for many years, operation has been done, first by plating the hindfoot to hold the scaphoid in position (Figs. XI.34 and XI.35) and, later, by replacement of the injured bone with a prosthetic insert. After these operations, the greyhounds often return to racing but without the same handicap as before.

A corollary to a stress fracture of the navicular bone is that a fracture of the calcaneus on the same side can occur. It may be a stress fracture that has become complete; it is difficult to compare this bone to that in the human since it is obvious that in the greyhound the calcaneus is subject to tremendous leverage quite unlike that in the human. It could, however, be compared to the olecranon, since the stresses are somewhat similar. Sometimes the calcaneal fracture occurs with that in the navicular bone, perhaps because it has already started a stress fracture, or because the shortening of the medial border of the foot causes greater strain on the calcaneus by increasing its leverage. As can be seen in Figure XI.36 internal fixation is used to allow the greyhound to live out its life with a satisfactory hindleg and to be used for stud purposes.

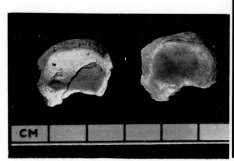

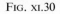

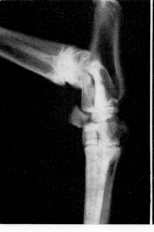

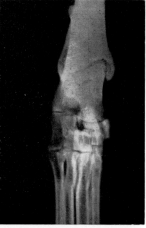

FIG. XI.30   FIG. XI.31   FIG. XI.32   FIG. XI.33

Figure XI.30 shows a dried specimen of a right navicular bone from a greyhound with an undisplaced stress fracture. Figure XI.31 shows a fresh specimen of a right navicular bone. The bruising of the articular cartilage is seen and this extends deeply within the bone.

Two radiographs of the ankle and foot of a greyhound who had sustained a stress fracture of the navicular bone. The displacement and consequent shortening of the medial border of the foot is well shown.

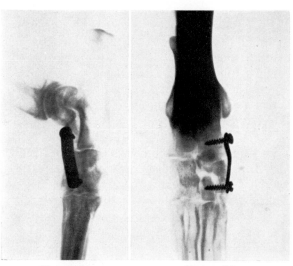

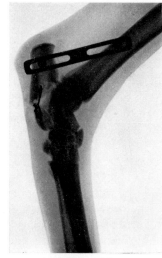

FIG. XI.34   FIG. XI.35   FIG. XI.36

Radiographs taken after open reduction and plating of the navicular bone.

Another possible stress fracture in the greyhound: while racing, the calcaneus can fracture, quite often in association with a navicular stress fracture. It also is treated by open operation. The plate is necessary as a start until the fracture is united, when it can be removed.

CHAPTER TWELVE

EPILOGUE

The description of stress fractures in this book is entirely from personal experience and has, throughout, been purely clinical. The writings of others have not been borrowed, nor has refuge been sought in references.

In this final chapter certain thoughts on the aetiology of stress fractures are given that seem acceptable on clinical grounds, and which may offer some slight help to the scientific research worker interested in bone strength and its failure. Also certain of the large number of papers on stress fractures are described; some omissions are deliberate, some are through lack of language and some are from the frailty of human endeavour.

Aetiology

A study of stress fractures over many years has given a certain understanding of the nature and strength of the living bone, in clinical practice, and if there is any particular fact that has been found to be of greater importance than another it is that living bone is only as strong as it needs to be for everyday activities. If activity is abruptly increased by necessity, will-power or simple *joie de vivre*, the muscles will increase in tone and produce stresses stronger than those which the bone can withstand and a stress fracture may occur in some people. The emphasis must be on the *abrupt increase* in exercise and muscle tone because, as the muscle increases in tone, the strength of the bone will also increase but not so fast; this is what makes the athlete who is starting training, or the services recruit, more liable to stress fractures than is the seasoned sportsman or serviceman.

Athletes are, by and large, extraordinarily fit and cannot be considered as a group to have any basic pathological abnormality. It is the occurrence of stress fractures in athletes that lends the greatest support to the definition that a stress fracture occurs in normal bone within a normal person. That children also are susceptible is important for, surely, were there to have been a bone abnormality, there would have been further development of that abnormality during the later years of growth; this has never been found. Bone disease can and does weaken bone; this will allow a true pathological fracture to occur (in passing, it is of great interest to observe that when the weakened bone begins to break the symptoms are identical to those of a stress fracture, for indeed that is what is occurring in the remaining bone adjacent to the lesion).

Many of the stress fractures described, as for example in the femoral neck or the tibia in elderly women, occur through osteoporotic bone; the latter is so common that, like baldness in men, it cannot be considered abnormal in the state of knowledge which we have at the moment because, with age, osteoporosis is expected in women and it is an unusual situation when it does not occur.

The amount of clinical, biochemical and astronautical research that has gone into trying to understand osteoporosis is very great. Perhaps the problem would be more quickly resolved were a strictly clinical approach to be used and certain signposts allowed to indicate the correct path to the solution. Stress fractures occur with great frequency in older women with osteoporosis. Stress fractures also occur in the most healthy young adults. The connection between the two is muscle tone and bone strength. When muscle strength increases so does bone strength, but less rapidly, thereby leaving the bone more susceptible to a stress fracture. The limb of a patient immobilised in plaster rapidly loses bone strength, but more rapidly loses muscle tone. If the latter is maintained by diligent exercise, so is the strength of the bone. Decubitus has the same effect because it immobilises the body as a whole so that the normal muscle tone needed for the erect posture is lost. Weightlessness is the extreme form of decubitus, with no tone required and practically no muscle effort to perform otherwise Herculean tasks. The normal skeletal frame was built for the muscles to withstand gravity, without which there is little need for a strong and rigid skeleton.

The process of ageing is inherent to the body: it is remorseless in its progress and starts, if the degeneration of articular cartilage is studied, in childhood well before growth has ceased. Ageing, therefore, is as much a physiological process as is the growth of the body; it is part of normal existence. The strength of bone and its internal structure and architecture will vary with growth—or age—but will be influenced at different times by the same stresses which show in different ways. In the child the appearance of the stress fractures that occur are, in many respects, different to those in the mature adult. The greenstick fracture in the child can in no way be considered pathological merely because the bone reacts differently from the adult, in whom a similar force and a similar injury produces the ordinary fracture. The stress fracture in the child often has its counterpart in the osteoporotic old lady—but much less often in the old man, who appears to lose bone strength no more rapidly than he does muscle tone. That the infant can have a stress fracture, when walking has barely started, suggests that the balance between bone strength and muscle power is delicate; particularly is this important because it is muscle power, and not weight or gravity, that causes a stress fracture.

With our present knowledge, therefore, it is not possible to accept that a stress fracture in an osteoporotic patient is a pathological fracture, so it can be included in an attempt to formulate, on a purely clinical basis, the aetiology of stress fractures. It has been suggested that the inception of the stress fracture is within the apatite crystal, and it has been shown that muscle power is responsible for the stress. But there is still to be answered the question: Why do some children, some athletes, some middle-aged people and some elderly women get stress fractures but not others?

No bone is stronger than it need be is also a finding. The athlete and services recruit build up muscle tone; bone strength increases but not so fast as the muscles and, with excessive training, stress fractures occur. If bone strength is to be maintained the athlete must stay in training. If he has even a short while off sport a stress fracture is much more likely to occur than otherwise, when training starts again.

In children and young adults the increase in bone strength follows increase in muscle strength; in late middle- and old-age muscle power decreases; with it decreases bone strength. Can osteoporosis be prevented, to the extent it occurs in the otherwise normal though ageing person, by maintaining muscle strength? That there is one simple cause

Q

for osteoporosis is unlikely but at least one of the many reasons is that the failure of muscle to maintain a strong tone allows the bone to weaken. Only when the full reasons for declining strength with age are understood may this one cause be prevented; perhaps it is not only of interest that men in the second half of life get far fewer stress fractures than women of the same age, but it is also a strong hint towards the understanding of aetiology.

Stress fractures in osteoporosis have a different pattern to those of the younger adult; but if osteoporosis is accepted as part of the physiological process of ageing, then it is possible on a clinical basis to consider an aetiology of stress fractures that will encompass all varieties seen at all ages.

The most important clinical finding is that a stress fracture occurs in normal bone with normal use; very often stress fractures are seen in the most healthy and fit persons, notably athletes, in whom there is no suggestion of general or local disease. Investigations and studies of biopsy material support this view.

Another finding is that there has been, preceding the stress fracture, some unusual, but not abnormal, activity which invariably has meant increased muscular activity, whether in the newly inducted recruit with a heavy training programme or in the older person who takes a walking holiday. Not all of the histories accounted by patients give this specific and obvious connection between increased use of the part involved and the stress fracture but the more that the connection is looked for the more it is found.

The common finding is increased muscular activity leading to a stress fracture because the bone in which the stress fracture occurs is not strong enough to withstand the increased stress. The extra weight consistent with intensive muscular activity, as seen in recruits, is at first an increase in muscle volume; only later do the bones show an increased strength although little by little and day by day their strength does increase but at a slower proportional rate to the muscle. The opposite also occurs: when activity ceases, muscles waste very rapidly but it seems also that the bone loses strength much faster than it is able to gain strength. Two or three weeks in a plaster is sufficient for the naked eye to see the decreased bone density in a radiograph—speedily when muscle activity in the part concerned has also been curtailed. When movement and tone in the muscles is maintained so is the bone strength. This is almost so well known that it hardly needs stating but it is very significant in the context of bone strength and muscular activity. The athlete, off sport for a few weeks, returns to training and is then liable to a stress fracture. This sequence of events is not at all uncommon.

Again, there is no difference in the overall effort in running on smooth grass or a hard pavement; yet the latter, by needing a more forceful muscle response to protect the footfall which is not cushioned by turf, increases the liability to a stress fracture. This may also play a part in the middle-aged lady who goes out on a day's shopping and sustains a stress fracture of the fibula; normally she may do as much walking around her house but not on hard pavements.

It may appear paradoxical to suggest that the weakening of muscle causes stress fractures in the patient who has simple osteoporosis. It is not, however, difficult to understand. With the decrease in overall strength of muscle, tone diminishes and osteoporosis increases because the bones need no longer preserve strength to withstand the forces no longer present. It is at this stage that any slight but reasonably rapid change in situation may upset the balance of bone strength and muscle tone: thus any cause of increased activity may develop the muscle tone—and strength—or some slight indisposition may cause enough lack of activity to increase the osteoporosis, even if only a very little. Any such imbalance can precipitate a stress fracture, as has been reiterated above in the athlete who stops training for only a short while. There is no need, therefore, to look further than simple physiology for the cause of the increased numbers of stress fractures in the older woman. This is not to say that were all women after the menopause exercised to the full osteoporosis would not occur, but it would certainly be diminished.

If the foregoing is accepted, and it seems difficult not to do so, then a stress fracture occurs in a bone unable to withstand the stresses imposed upon it, and not that the bone is fatigued by some inherent condition or change. Such change as occurs is brought about by the bone being stressed by the pull of the muscles.

Bone is living with an abundant blood supply. Were the latter not to be used or necessary it would not be there. Bone metabolism might not be high in one sense, but it needs a continuous flow of fresh blood to service the bone crystals that preserve the hardness of the bone and, with the collagen fibres, its strength. If the apatite crystals in the Haversian systems, which make up osteons, are to withstand the everyday forces used upon them, they must be continually refreshed because, in absorbing energy, denaturing of the crystalline structure occurs. This denaturing occurs also in inert materials such as cast-iron, in which the crystals alter with vibration or intermittent stresses to allow the metal to become brittle and fail in strength.

There is no difficulty in understanding the development of a stress fracture once the initial cellular failure has occurred. It is the cause of that first minute lesion that has to be understood; why should the apatite crystals fail, probably as a small group rather than as one alone?

It has been shown that, in the common stress fractures particular sites are affected. In the fibula this is just above the lateral malleolus where, with normal muscular contraction, the greatest bend in the bone occurs. It is also clear that, because of the different muscles used, different forms of usage of a limb will induce different stresses on the bone concerned with a distinct type of stress fracture for each: this is well exemplified by the runner and the ballet dancer, one with the oblique stress fracture low down on the tibia and the other with the transverse fracture across the middle of the shaft. At these sites the stresses imposed on the bone are the greatest; it is not chance that the fibula can be shown to be bent by simple muscle power at the level where its stress fractures are usually to be found. At these sites the bone, overstressed by the muscular activity, develops the clinical stress fracture. The cause of the weakening must be a failure of the apatite crystals within the osteon, which have been denatured so quickly either because there were too few crystals to absorb the energy or because the renaturing of each crystal took too long because of inadequate nutrition. When one crystal too many has been denatured, the strength of that osteon is lost and a physical, if microscopical break, or solution of continuity within the bone, will occur. Once this has happened the whole process of a physical inflammation occurs, with its increase in blood supply and the further weakening of the bone that this entails.

Much of what has been said is conjecture; nevertheless the conjecture is based on clinical observation. A great deal of experimental work needs to be done to demonstrate the truth—and only a little has been done so far because it is only by the study of the reaction of living bone to stress that the answers will be found.

Studies in the Literature

There have been many workers interested in stress fractures over many years. A thorough study of the literature adds to the understanding of stress fractures, but not everything written is correct. Therefore a vast and unselected bibliography is of little value.

It is probable that the first clinical description of a stress fracture was made in 1855 by a German military surgeon called Breithaupt. For a good report of this see Devan and Carlton (1954). In 1773 Gooch had given a good description of a cough fracture which makes fascinating reading. Stechow in 1897 is credited by Haggart and Eberle (1956) to have given the first description of a radiograph of a march fracture. Lane in 1855 described some points in the physiology and pathology of the bone skeleton produced by pressure, and in 1917 Koch published his laws of bone architecture. Looser described his zones in 1920, and Milkman described multiple spontaneous idiopathic symmetrical fractures in 1934. An important work was that of Aleman in 1929, who appears to have understood very well stress and its effect on bone.

The strength of bone in regard to its fatigue life has been described by Evans and Riolo in 1970, and osteoporosis and its relationship to stress fractures by Devas (1967a). In recent years there has also been much interest in avascular necrosis of the femoral head and Perthes' disease; it is almost impossible in clinical writings to separate the two, particularly when the aetiology, as opposed to the clinical course, is studied. Before any reading is done on this subject the anatomy of the femoral head must be understood. The description by Trueta and Harrison (1953) has become a classical anatomical study. Before this, in 1939, Freund had studied osteochondritic diseases of the hip; Ratliff (1962) had studied the problem in Perthes' disease. In 1964 Merle d'Aubigné drew attention to the grave problem of idiopathic avascular necrosis of the hip in adults, as did Hastings and Macnab in 1965 with a special regard to steroid arthropathy. Since then there has been a considerable investigation into this condition in both the adult and child and experimentally in animals. As will have been seen from this book, avascularity of the femoral head can follow from a stress fracture within the head (Kemp, 1968, 1969; Rosingh and James, 1969; Stougard, 1969; Zahir and Freeman, 1972; Sanchis, Zahir and Freeman, 1973; Solomon, 1973.)

On the experimental and microscopic stress fracture there have been works by Evans and Riolo (1970), Freeman, Day and Swanson (1971), Griffiths, Swanson and Freeman (1971) and Todd, Freeman and Pirie (1972). Braddock in 1959 did some experimental work in connection with Freiberg's infraction.

White, Protheroe, Glennie and Jackson (1969) showed that post-irradiation fractures of the femoral neck were most probably caused by the vascular damage.

Before passing on to specific stress fractures there are many good papers on the subject in general, such as Ollonquist (1937), Camp and McCullough (1941), Hartley (1943), Nickerson (1943), Bertram (1944), Robin and Thompson (1944), Leveton (1946), Devas (1963), Pentecost, Murray and Brindley (1964), Gilbert and Johnson (1966); the book by Morris and Blickenstaff (1967) has a vast quantity of references.

Discussions on steroid treatment and its effect on bone have been described by Rosenberg (1958), Bernstein and Freyberg (1961), Hader and Storey (1962), Velayos, Leidholt, Smyth and Priest (1966).

Miller, Markheim and Towbin in 1967 described multiple stress fractures in rheumatoid arthritis. Morris in 1966 described a stress fracture in an arthrodesed hip, and a study of biopsies from stress fractures was made in 1963 by Johnson, Stradford, Geis, Dineen and Kerley. In 1959 Swiderski published a monograph putting forward the view that the new bone formation on the surface of the tibia was a form of avulsion of the periosteum.

The Fibula

Burrows in 1940 and again in 1948 gave excellent descriptions of this stress fracture and quoted Siemens (1942) as having described a 16-month-old child with a stress fracture of the central shaft of the fibula, but the original paper has not been traced. In 1952 Griffiths described stress fractures of the fibula in children, and other workers include Ingersoll (1943) and Devas and Sweetnam (1956 and 1958). In 1944 Lord and Coutts described a fracture in the upper third of the fibula occurring in parachutists.

The Tibia

In 1956 Burrows described the transverse stress fracture of the tibia in ballet dancers and pointed out that it was a dangerous condition. Previously, Ollonquist (1929) had described stress fractures of the tibia, and Roberts and Vogt (1939) and Nordentoft (1940) also gave good descriptions. In 1945 Wolfe and Robertson provided a good review of the literature on stress fractures of the tibia and femur. Singer and Maudsley in 1954 described stress fractures in the lower third of the tibia which were transverse and of the compression type. Other papers include Murray (1957), Devas (1960a), Wheeldon (1961), Maudsley (1963) and Reynolds (1972) described stress fractures in the shin with knee deformities above. Devas (1958) lists most of the earlier references needed for further study. Freidenberg (1971) reported on two transverse stress fractures on which biopsy was done with the inevitable result of a great delay in union.

The Femur

The anatomy of the blood supply of the head of the femur described by Trueta and Harrison in 1953 has been specially mentioned to understand how any injury within the head can block off the blood supply. Burrows in 1940 described a stress fracture in a femoral neck with coxa vara, and other works include those of Hansson (1938), Miller (1950), Haggart and Eberle (1956) Mankin and Bower (1960), Jeffery (1962), Linscheid and Coventry (1962), Ernst (1964) and Devas (1965). Stress fractures in the shaft of the femur are also described by Peterson (1942), Kroenig and Shelton (1963), Provost and Morris (1969) and, in 'joggers', Graham (1970); Grundy (1970) has described the femoral shaft fractures in Paget's disease.

The Patella

Reference should be made to Sinding-Larsen (1921), Johansson (1922) and Hawley and Griswold (1928) for 'osteochondritis' but there are few published articles on stress fractures of the patella; Devas in 1960(b), had found no previous description of the lesion.

The Pelvis

In 1963 Byers described, with biopsy studies, ischiopubic osteochondritis, a condition of the pelvis seen in children resembling stress fractures which are detailed by Devas

(1963). Other descriptions of stress fractures of the pelvis were given in 1943 by Jones and in 1954 by Selakovich and Love. Gschwend, in 1967, described three ischiopubic stress fractures after arthrodesis of the hip.

The Foot

Robert Jones, in 1902, described a fracture of the fifth metatarsal bone, probably from stress. Hullinger in 1944 described calcaneal fractures; also good accounts were given by Leabhart in 1959 and Darby in 1967. Some other papers of note on the march fracture include Childress (1943), Bernstein and Stone (1944), Carlson and Wertz (1944), Krause and Thompson (1944), Bernstein, Childress, Fox, Archer and Stone (1946), Macpherson (1951), Devan and Carlton (1954), Smillie (1957) and North (1966). In 1960 Golding described the stress fracture in the sesamoid. Towne, Blazina and Cozen (1970) described the navicular stress fracture and Savoca's (1971) paper includes stress fractures of one talus and one first metatarsal. Waugh in 1958 described the ossification and blood supply of the navicular bone in relation to Köhler's disease.

The Arm and Trunk

There are few references to true stress fractures of the humerus but papers of interest include Wilmoth (1930), Herzmark and Klune (1952), Bingham (1959) and Brogdon and Crow (1960). Stress fractures of the ulna have been described by Evans in 1955 and, earlier, in 1948 by Kitchin. Waris in 1946 and Miller in 1960 described javelin throwers' injuries. There are several papers on one specific case of a 'stress' fracture of the capitate bone but this is a good example of not accepting all that is in the literature as true. Reference should be made to Newman in 1963 for the aetiology of spondylolisthesis as it should to Henderson (1966); other works include those of Hadley (1955), Johnson and Southwick (1960) and Harris and Wiley (1963). Horner in 1964 described stress fractures of the lower ribs.

Stress Avulsions

Avulsion of the ischial epiphysis has been described by Barnes and Hinds (1972) and by Schlonsky and Olix also in 1972. Of the patients described by Hand, Hand and Dunn in 1971, at least some had true stress avulsions of the tibial tubercle.

Comparative Stress Fractures

The papers referring to the greyhound are Bateman (1958, 1959 and 1963) and Devas (1961); to the horse, Devas (1967b), and much help on the subject of horses has been obtained from Mr P. J. Davidson (1967) and Professor F. J. Milne (1966).

In the foregoing pages of this book an attempt has been made to collate the various stress fractures at various sites. Deliberately no attempt has been made to deal with specific groups of patients, such as athletes, because the stress fractures that can occur in any particular group of people should be diagnosed and treated against the background of a sound knowledge of the behaviour of the living bone and its reaction to stress in the normal person.

References

ALEMAN, O. (1929) Omsk marchschalst (syndesmites metatarsea). *Tidskrift i Militar Halsovard*, **54**, 191–208.

BARNES, S. T. & HINDS, R. B. (1972) Pseudotumour of the ischium. A late manifestation of avulsion of the ischial epiphysis. *Journal of Bone and Joint Surgery*, **54-A**, 645.

BATEMAN, J. K. (1958) Broken hock in the greyhound: repair methods and the plastic scaphoid. *Veterinary Record*, **70**, 621.

BATEMAN, J. K. (1959) Fractured sesamoids in the greyhound. *Veterinary Record*, **71**, 101.

BATEMAN, J. K. (1963) Repair of fractured right os calcis in the racing greyhound. *Veterinary Record*, **75**, 1,001–3.

BERNSTEIN, A., CHILDRESS, M. A., FOX, K. W., ARCHER, M. C. & STONE, J. R. (1946) March fractures of the foot. *American Journal of Surgery*, **71**, 355.

BERNSTEIN, C. A. & FREYBERG, F. H. (1961) Rheumatoid patients after five or more years of cortico-steroid treatment: a comparative analysis of 183 cases. *Annals of Internal Medicine*, **54**, 938.

BERNSTEIN, A. & STONE, J. R. (1944) March fracture. *Journal of Bone and Joint Surgery*, **26**, 743.

BERTRAM, D. R. (1944) 'Stress' fracture of bone. *British Journal of Radiology*, **17**, 257.

BINGHAM, E. L. (1959) Fractures of the humerus from muscular violence. *U.S. Armed Forces Medical Journal*, **10**, 22.

BRADDOCK, F. T. F. (1959) Experimental epiphysial injury and Freiberg's disease. *Journal of Bone and Joint Surgery*, **41-B**, 154.

BREITHAUPT (1855). Zur Pathologie des Menschlichen Fusses. *Med. Zeitung, Berlin*, **24**, 169.

BROGDON, B. G. & CROW, N. E. (1960) Little leaguer's elbow. *American Journal of Roentgenology*, **83**, 671.

BURROWS, H. J. (1940) Spontaneous fracture of the apparently normal fibula in its lowest third. *British Journal of Surgery*, **28**, 82.

BURROWS, H. J. (1940) Incomplete fracture of femoral neck in a case of infantile coxa vara. *British Medical Journal*, i, 569.

BURROWS, H. J. (1948) Fatigue fractures of the fibula. *Journal of Bone and Joint Surgery*, **30-B**, 266.

BURROWS, H. J. (1950) Fatigue infraction of the middle of the tibia in ballet dancers. *Journal of Bone and Joint Surgery*, **38-B**, 83.

BYERS, P. D. (1963) Ischiopubic 'osteochondritis'. *Journal of Bone and Joint Surgery*, **45-B**, 694.

CAMP, J. D. & McCULLOUGH, J. A. L. (1941) Pseudofractures in diseases affecting the skeletal system. *Radiology*, **36**, 651.

CARLSON, O. D. & WERTZ, R. F. (1944) March fractures including others than those of the foot. *Radiology*, **43**, 48.

CHILDRESS, H. M. (1943) March fractures of the lower extremity. Report of a case of march fracture of a cuneiform bone. *War Medicine*, **4**, 152.

DARBY, R. E. (1967) Stress fractures of the os calcis. *Journal of the American Medical Association*, **200**, 1183.

DAVIDSON, P. J. (1967) Personal communication.

DEVAN, W. T. & CARLTON, D. C. (1954) The march fracture persists. *American Journal of Surgery*, **87**, 227.

DEVAS, M. B. (1958) Stress fractures of the tibia in athletes or shin soreness. *Journal of Bone and Joint Surgery*, **40-B**, 227.

DEVAS, M. B. (1960a) Stress fractures of the patella. *Journal of Bone and Joint Surgery*, **42-B**, 71.

DEVAS, M. B. (1960b) Longitudinal stress fractures: another variety seen in long bones. *Journal of Bone and Joint Surgery*, **42-B**, 508.

DEVAS, M. B. (1961) Compression stress fractures in man and the greyhound. *Journal of Bone and Joint Surgery*, **43-B**, 540.

DEVAS, M. B. (1963) Stress fractures in children. *Journal of Bone and Joint Surgery*, **45-B**, 528.

DEVAS, M. B. (1965) Stress fractures of the femoral neck. *Journal of Bone and Joint Surgery*, **47-B**, 728.

DEVAS, M. B. (1967a) Osteoporosis. *Transactions of the Medical Society of London*, **83**, 180.

DEVAS, M. B. (1967b) Shin splints or stress fractures of the metacarpal bone in horses, and shin soreness, or stress fractures of the tibia, in man. *Journal of Bone and Joint Surgery*, **49-B**, 310.

DEVAS, M. B. & SWEETNAM, D. R. (1958) Runner's fracture. *Practitioner*, **180**, 340.

DEVAS, M. B. & SWEETNAM, D. R. (1956) Stress fractures of the fibula. A review of 50 cases in athletes. *Journal of Bone and Joint Surgery*, **38-B**, 818.

ERNST, J. (1964) Stress fracture of the neck of the femur. *Journal of Trauma*, **4**, 71.

EVANS, D. L. (1955) Fatigue fracture of the ulna. *Journal of Bone and Joint Surgery*, **37-B**, 618.

EVANS, F. G. & RIOLO, M. L. (1970) Relations between the fatigue life and histology of adult human cortical bone. *Journal of Bone and Joint Surgery*, **52-A**, 1579.

FREEMAN, M. A. R., DAY, W. H. & SWANSON, S. A. V. (1971) Fatigue fracture in the subchondral bone of the human cadaver femoral head. *Medical and Biological Engineering*, **9**, 619.

FREUND, E. (1939) Osteochondritis dissecans. Femoral head. *Archives of Surgery*, **39**, 323.

FRIEDENBERG, Z. B. (1971) Fatigue fractures of the tibia. *Clinical Orthopaedics*, **76**, 111–115.

GILBERT, R. S. & JOHNSON, H. A. (1966) Stress fractures in military recruits—a review of 12 years' experience. *Military Medicine*, **131**, 716–721.

GOLDING, C. (1960) Museum pages. V: The sesamoids of the hallux. *Journal of Bone and Joint Surgery*, **42-B**, 840.

GOOCH, B. (1773) *Medical and Chirurgical Observations, as an Appendix to a Former Publication.* G. Robinson. Page 55. Description of a cough fracture.

GRAHAM, C. E. (1970) Stress fractures in joggers. *Texas Medical Journal*, **66**, 68–73.

GRIFFITHS, A. L. (1952) Fatigue fracture of the fibula in childhood. *Archives of Diseases of Childhood.* **27**, 552.

GRIFFITHS, W. E. G., SWANSON, S. A. V. & FREEMAN, M. A. R. (1971) Experimental fatigue fracture of the human cadaveric femoral neck. *Journal of Bone and Joint Surgery*, **53-B**, 136.

GRUNDY, M. (1970) Fractures of the femur in Paget's disease of bone. *Journal of Bone and Joint Surgery*, **52-B**, 252.

GSCHWEND, N. (1967) Three ischiopubic fractures after arthrodesed hip. *Archiv orthopädische und Unfallchirurgie*, **62**, 363–367.

HADER, R. & STOREY, G. (1962) Spontaneous fractures in rheumatoid arthritis. *British Medical Journal*, ii, 1514.

HADLEY, L. A. (1955) Fatigue fracture of the fifth lumbar neural arch. Is spondylolysis a stress fracture? *Clinical Orthopaedics*, **6**, 110.

HAGGART, G. E. & EBERLE, H. J. (1956) Bilateral stress fractures of the neck of the femur. *Lahey Clinic Bulletin*, **10**, 15.

HAND, W. L., HAND, C. R. & DUNN, A. W. (1971) Avulsion fractures of the tibial tubercle. *Journal of Bone and Joint Surgery*, **53-A**, 1579.

HANSSON, C. J. (1938) On insufficiency fractures of femur and tibia. *Acta radiologica*, **19**, 554.

HARRIS, R. I. & WILEY, J. J. (1963) Acquired spondylolysis as a sequel to spine fusion. *Journal of Bone and Joint Surgery*, **48-A**, 1159.

HARTLEY, J. B. (1943) 'Stress' or 'fatigue' fractures in bone. *British Journal of Radiology*, **16**, 255.

HASTINGS, D. E. & MACNAB, I. (1965) Spontaneous avascular necrosis of the femoral head. *Canadian Journal of Surgery*, **8**, 68–83.

HAWLEY, G. W. & GRISWOLD, A. S. (1928) Larsen Johansson's disease of the patella. *Surgery, Gynaecology and Obstetrics*, **47**, 68.

HENDERSON, E. D. (1966) Results of surgical treatment of spondylolisthesis. *Journal of Bone and Joint Surgery*, **48-A**, 616.

HERZMARK, M. H. & KLUNE, F. R. (1952) Ball-throwing fracture of the humerus. *Medical Annals of the District of Columbia*, **21**, 196.

HORNER, D. B. (1964) Lumbar back pain arising from stress fractures of the lower ribs. *Journal of Bone and Joint Surgery*, **46-A**, 1553.

HULLINGER, C. W. (1944) Insufficiency fracture of the calcaneus similar to march fracture of metatarsal. *Journal of Bone and Joint Surgery*, **26**, 751.

INGERSOLL, C. F. (1943) Ice skater's fracture. *American Journal of Roentgenology*, **50**, 469.

JEFFERY, C. C. (1962) Spontaneous fractures of the femoral neck. *Journal of Bone and Joint Surgery*, **44-B**, 543.

JOHANSSON, S. (1922) Eine bischer nicht beschriebene. Krankheit der Patella. *Hygiei*, **84**, 161.

JOHNSON, J. T. H. & SOUTHWICK, W. O. (1960) Bone growth after spine fusion: a clinical survey. *Journal of Bone and Joint Surgery*, **42-A**, 1396.

JOHNSON, L. C., STRADFORD, H. T., GEIS, R. W., DINEEN, J. R. & KERLEY, E. (1963) Histogenesis of stress fractures. *Journal of Bone and Joint Surgery*, **45-A**, 1542.

JONES, D. B. (1943) March fracture of the inferior pubic ramus. *Radiology*, **41**, 586.

JONES, R. (1902) Fracture of the fifth metatarsal bone. *Liverpool Medico-Chirurgical Journal*, **22**, 103.

KEMP, H. (1968) Experimental Perthes' disease. *Journal of Bone and Joint Surgery*, **50-B**, 233.

KEMP, H. B. S. (1968) Avascular necrosis of the femoral head in dogs. *Journal of Bone and Joint Surgery*, **50-B**, 431.

KEMP, H. B. S. (1969) Experimental Perthes' disease. *Journal of Bone and Joint Surgery*, **51-B**, 178.

KITCHIN, I. D. (1948) Fatigue fracture of the ulna. *Journal of Bone and Joint Surgery*, **30-B**, 622.

KOCH, J. C. (1917) The laws of bone architecture. *American Journal of Anatomy*, **21**, 177.

KRAUSE, G. R. & THOMPSON, J. R. (1944) An analysis of 200 cases. *American Journal of Roentgenology*, **52**, 281.

KROENING, P. M. & SHELTON, M. L. (1963) Stress fractures. *American Journal of Roentgenology*, **89**, 1281.

LANE, W. A. (1855) Some points in the physiology and pathology of the changes produced by pressure in the bony skeleton of the trunk and shoulder girdle. *Guy's Hospital Reports*, **43**, 321.

LEABHART, J. W. (1959) Stress fractures of the calcaneus. *Journal of Bone and Joint Surgery*, **41-A**, 1285.

LEVETON, A. L. (1946) March (fatigue) fractures of the long bones of the lower extremity and pelvis. *American Journal of Surgery*, **71**, 222.

LINSCHEID, R. L. & COVENTRY, M. B. (1962) Unrecognised fractures of long bones suggesting primary bone tumours. *Proceedings Mayo Clinic*, **37**, 599.

LOOSER, E. (1920) *Zentralblatt für Chirurgie*, **47**, 1470.

LORD, C. D. & COUTTS, J. W. (1944) A study of typical parachute injuries occurring in 250,000 jumps at the parachute school. *Journal of Bone and Joint Surgery*, **26**, 547.

MacPHERSON, D. A. (1951) Stress fractures of metatarsal in childhood. *British Medical Journal*, ii, 339.

MANKIN, H. J. & BOWER, T. D. (1960) Bilateral idiopathic aseptic necrosis of the femur in adults. *Journal of the Hospital for Joint Diseases*, **23**, 42.

MAUDSLEY, R. H. (1963) Fatigue fractures of both tibia and fibula. *Postgraduate Medical Journal*, **36**, 650.

MERLE D'AUBIGNÉ, R. (1964) Non-traumatic aseptic necrosis of the femoral head. *Journal of Bone and Joint Surgery*, **46-B**, 161.

MILKMAN, L. A. (1934) Multiple spontaneous idiopathic symmetrical fractures. *American Journal of Radiology*, **32**, 622.

MILLER, B., MARKHEIM, H. R. & TOWBIN, M. N. (1967) Multiple stress fractures in rheumatoid arthritis. *Journal of Bone and Joint Surgery*, **49-A**, 1408.

MILLER, J. E. (1960) Javelin thrower's elbow. *Journal of Bone and Joint Surgery*, **42-B**, 788.

MILLER, L. F. (1950) Bilateral stress fracture of the neck of the femur. *Journal of Bone and Joint Surgery*, **32-A**, 695.

MILNE, F. J. (1966) Personal communication.

MORRIS, J. B. (1966) Charnley compression arthrodesis of the hip. *Journal of Bone and Joint Surgery*, **48-B**, 260.

MORRIS, J. M. & BLICKENSTAFF, L. D. (1967) *Fatigue Fractures: A Clinical Study*. Charles C. Thomas: Springfield, Illinois.

MURRAY, D. S. (1957) Fatigue fractures of the lower tibia and fibula in the same leg. *Journal of Bone and Joint Surgery*, **39-B**, 302.

NEWMAN, P. H. (1963) The aetiology of spondylolisthesis. *Journal of Bone and Joint Surgery*, **45-B**, 39.

NICKERSON, S. H. (1943) March fracture, or insufficiency fracture. *American Journal of Surgery*, **62**, 154.

NORDENTOFT, J. M. (1940) Some cases of soldier's fracture. *Acta radiologica*, **21**, 615.

NORTH, A. F. JUN. (1966) Bilateral symmetrical march fractures simulating juvenile rheumatoid arthritis. *Arthritis and Rheumatism*, **9**, 77.

OLLONQUIST, L. J. (1929) Callus formation without fracture of shin bones. *Duodecim*, **45**, 473.

OLLONQUIST, L. J. (1937) Osteopathia itineraria tibiae. *Acta radiologica*, **18**, 526.

PENTECOST, R. L., MURRAY, R. A. & BRINDLEY, H. H. (1964) Fatigue, insufficiency and pathological fractures. *Journal of the American Medical Association*, **187**, 1001.

PETERSON, L. T. (1942) March fracture of the femur. *Journal of Bone and Joint Surgery*, **24**, 184.

PROVOST, R. A. & MORRIS, J. M. (1969) Fatigue fracture of the femoral shaft. *Journal of Bone and Joint Surgery*, **51-A**, 487.

RATLIFF, A. H. C. (1962) Avascular necrosis of the head of the femur after fractures of the femoral neck in children and Perthes' disease. *Proceedings of the Royal Society of Medicine*, **55**, 504.

REYNOLDS, M. T. (1972) Stress fractures of the tibia in the elderly associated with knee deformity. *Proceedings of the Royal Society of Medicine*, **65**, 377–380.

ROBERTS, S. M. & VOGT, E. C. (1939) Pseudofracture of the tibia. *Journal of Bone and Joint Surgery*, **21**, 891.

ROBIN, P. A. & THOMPSON, S. B. (1944) Fatigue fractures. *Journal of Bone and Joint Surgery*, **26**, 557.

ROSENBERG, E. F. (1958) Rheumatoid arthritis: osteoporosis and fractures related to steroid therapy. *Acta medica Scandinavica*, Supplement 162.

ROSINGH, G. E. & JAMES, J. (1969) Early phases of avascular necrosis of the femoral head in rabbits. *Journal of Bone and Joint Surgery*, **51-B**, 165.

SANCHIS, M., ZAHIR, A. & FREEMAN, M. A. R. (1973) The experimental simulation of Perthes' disease by consecutive interruptions of the blood supply to the capital femoral epiphysis in the puppy. *Journal of Bone and Joint Surgery*, **55-A**, 335.

SAVOCA, C. J. (1971) Stress fractures. A classification of the earliest radiographic signs. *Radiology*, **100**, 519–524.

SCHLONSKY, J. & OLIX, M. L. (1972) Functional disability following avulsion fracture of the ischial epiphysis. *Journal of Bone and Joint Surgery*, **54-A**, 641.

SELAKOVICH, W. & LOVE, L. (1954) Stress fractures of the pubic ramus. *Journal of Bone and Joint Surgery*, **36-A**, 573.

SIEMENS, W. (1942) Frakturen der Umbauzonen aus der fibula im Anschluss an besondere Sportliche Beausprachung. *Zentralblatt für Chirurgie*, **60**, 2739.

SINDING-LARSEN, M. F. (1921) A hitherto unknown affection of the patella in children. *Acta radiologica*, **1**, 171.

SINGER, M. & MAUDSLEY, R. H. (1954) Fatigue fractures of the lower tibia. *Journal of Bone and Joint Surgery*, **36-B**, 647.

SMILLIE, I. S. (1957) Freiberg's infraction. *Journal of Bone and Joint Surgery*, **39-B**, 580.

SOLOMON, L. (1973) Drug-induced arthropathy and necrosis of the femoral head. *Journal of Bone and Joint Surgery*, **55-B**, 246.

STECHOW (1897) Fussödem und Rontgenstrahlen. *Deutsche Militärärztliche Zeitschrift*, **26**, 465.

STOUGARD, J. (1969) Post-traumatic avascular necrosis of the femoral head in children. *Journal of Bone and Joint Surgery*, **51-B**, 354.

STUBBS, G. (1766) *The Anatomy of the Horse.* (Reprinting of the plates with a modern paraphrase by J. C. McCann and C. W. Ottaway, London, Hill, 1938.)

SWIDERSKI, G. (1959) *Hyperporosis Osteomuscularis Crisis.* Poznan.

TODD, R. C., FREEMAN, M. A. R. & PIRIE, C. J. (1972) Isolated trabecular fatigue fractures in the femoral head. *Journal of Bone and Joint Surgery*, **54-B**, 723.

TOWNE, L. C., BLAZINA, M. E. & COZEN, L. N. (1970) Fatigue fracture of the tarsal navicular. *Journal of Bone and Joint Surgery*, **52-A**, 376.

TRUETA, J. & HARRISON, M. H. M. (1953) The normal vascular anatomy of the femoral head in adult man. *Journal of Bone and Joint Surgery*, **35-B**, 442.

VELAYOS, E. E., LEIDHOLT, J. D., SMYTH, C. J. & PRIEST, R. (1966) Arthropathy associated with steroid therapy. *Annals of Internal Medicine*, **64**, 759.

WARIS, W. (1946) Elbow injuries of javelin throwers. *Acta chirurgica scandinavica*, **93**, 563.

WAUGH, W. (1958) The ossification and vascularisation of the tarsal navicular and their relation to Köhler's disease. *Journal of Bone and Joint Surgery*, **40-B**, 765.

WHEELDON, F. T. (1961) Spontaneous fractures of the shin in the presence of knee deformities. *Proceedings of the Royal Society of Medicine*, **54**, 1108.

WHITE, J., PROTHEROE, K., GLENNIE, J. & JACKSON, W. (1969) The aetiology and treatment of post-irradiation fractures of the femoral neck. *Journal of Bone and Joint Surgery*, **51-B**, 569.

WILMOTH, C. L. (1930) Recurrent fracture of the humerus due to sudden extreme muscular action. *Journal of Bone and Joint Surgery*, **12**, 168.

WOLFE, H. R. I. & ROBERTSON, J. M. (1945) Fatigue fracture of femur and tibia. *Lancet*, ii, 11.

ZAHIR, A. & FREEMAN, M. A. R. (1972) Cartilage changes following a single episode of infarction of the capital femoral epiphysis in the dog. *Journal of Bone and Joint Surgery*, **54-A**, 125.

INDEX

Printed by T. & A Constable Ltd., Edinburgh